Cover Design: Mateus Rocha de Carvalho

MINDFULNESS

LESSONS TO LEARN
BEFORE GOING TO BED

To the main sources of my inspiration:

My family,

My friends,

My colleagues,

My patients.

|CONTENTS|

| ACKNOWLEDGEMENTS |

Thanks to my wonderful passion for the medical profession, the writing of this book became a marvelous adventure filled with numerous encounters and surprises; and it was all for you!

I am grateful to a lot of people, all of whom were deeply involved in one way or the other in the publication of this book. I am thankful to all who helped me by participating, by supporting me and in being a part of this project. Your involvement and your support are my motivation to continue writing and sharing ideas with the readers. Indeed, there are many who supported me, and I thank you all from the bottom of my heart!

Without any doubt, I was really fortunate to have you by my side!

My heartfelt gratitude to my family, friends, colleagues, as well as the entire community on meditation in compassion for all your help, company and participation!

| INTRODUCTION |

Imagine reading a book to help you fall asleep.... Did you know that your mind is most relaxed at the time you prepare to go to bed? This is also the moment when it is at its most receptive state and best able to assimilate information. Your night will end up disturbed and cumbersome if you go to sleep weighed down by the burdens of daily life.

On the other hand, your sleep will be peaceful and you will be well rested if you go to bed with a light head. The main aim of this book is thus to offer you short, simple stories and tales that will help you to forget for a moment the stresses of the world, from others, as well as your own.

Dear reader, the purpose of these tales is to take you back to experiences that, due to the demands of modern life, are most of the time pushed to the back of the mind.

Deliberate efforts have been made for the positive impacts of this book to be as close to our real lives as possible: the fears, all sorts of temptations, including the burdens of daily life that hang over our shoulders. There is always this quiet inner voice that does not leave us at peace.

To sum it up, there are so many underlying mental processes that contribute to the “rot” in our lives.

Fortunately, there are many positive illustrations for giving the mind a state of calm and tranquility, and which have enabled us to better understand these processes that otherwise would tear us apart.

****

The 69 short stories in this book have been divided into seven topics for you to reflect upon as you go to sleep. At the same time, they act as an appropriate safety valve in our lives:

- Impartiality: these stories bring out the power of observation in us, our ability to look at our inner selves and our own actions, with the aim of gradually establishing a sense of freedom in our lives.

- Patience: this is a necessary virtue to embrace if we wish to achieve inner well-being and tranquility.

- Fresh mind: ways to help you adapt to the pressures of life and to develop a mindset that can help you accept all manner of life's challenges.

- Confidence: confidence and self-respect are indispensable characteristics to help you rediscover your inner self beyond the views and opinions of others.

- No effort, no expectations: We spend our daily lives struggling against the realities of the world. We have our "demands", which we go to great lengths to achieve. Are there no other ways of finding happiness?

- Acceptance: our minds twist reality to make it conform to what we desire. Indeed, we always reject those things that are not in line with our desires.

- Thinking and letting go: this is about accepting the fact that our minds and feelings are ever-conscious as we pursue our daily activities. It would be possible for us to reduce our burdens once we accept this reality.

****

These topics are the seven pillars that help us to achieve a more comfortable and compassionate life. This fact about "compassion" is very fundamental, given that it operates as a sort of a release button to our inner selves and gives us the opportunity to escape from the hassles that make us worry and suffer. That is the power of Compassion.

These tales are anchored on wise sayings that have been in existence for ages. They have survived over the centuries, and this has given them a universal nature. On the one hand, they make a lot of sense, and on the other, they bring out in us a keen sense of observation.

The intention is that they should bring into the open the spontaneous actions that have a negative impact on our sleep and affect our daily lives. We can then deal with these factors once we become conscious of their existence. The first step is to carefully read the stories, right before going to sleep.

To get the most out of this book, it is strongly recommended that you read only one story per night, as you prepare to go to bed.

The question is: why just before going to bed? Well, it is at this time that your mind is best poised and suited to fully internalize the stories. They may appear ordinary, but their ability to transform your mind should not be under-estimated.

After reading one story at night, it would be important to give it time to develop within you. They are certainly very easy to understand, but they have in them very deep messages that unravel in you bit by bit. That is where the secret lies, the magic of Compassion: these tales will leave an impression, become real and capture your minds even when you are asleep. It is a slow, progressive and continuous process of infusion and development.

It would thus be important to fully internalize these stories. You should not be in a hurry to go on to the next story, it would be wise to exercise patience and proceed in a systematic manner. You can also expeditiously read the book over and over several times. You could equally refer back to a story that particularly touched your senses more than the rest (after completing the first reading of the entire book). I wish you happy reading! May these tales bring you good health, peace, and expose in the open the hidden obstacles in your inner selves.

| 1 |

| LIVING YOUR FEELINGS |

IMPARTIALITY

"The wise come up with new ideas,
fools spread them".

Heinrich Heine

A long time ago a certain wise man decided to confine himself in a cave, and vowed not come out until he had completely managed to control his feelings. People would look at him from afar and admire him, even though they considered him to be a sort of a hermit-saint.

Several years later, all alone in the cave and spending the better part of his time meditating, he finally managed to completely control his feelings. Indeed, his separation from the real world was so total that he did not have any feelings at all by the end of his life. He had even practically forgotten his own name.

He felt proud that he had achieved his aim, believing that he had lived a saintly life, and also that he had discovered the secret of wisdom.

However, on his deathbed in the cave, his mind was flooded with a lot of regrets: "There's so much I haven't done yet, so much joy that I've missed! Alas! It's too late now".

As he breathed his last, he finally understood that wisdom does not mean rejecting one's feelings, but rather acknowledging and being conscious of them as well.

Do you live your feelings or do you spend your time chasing after life's negative things?

| 2 |

| THE BUSY MAN |

THE VIRTUES OF PATIENCE

"Steadfast calm, availability at all timesl, multiple interests, are all true masters of the moment, given that they can take a back seat, through the use of humor".

Jean-Louis Servan-Schreiber

An old man is taking a stroll along the corridors of an old people's home, with the aid of a walking stick: he stops by a clock and takes a deep breath in desperation. When he was younger, he was an energetic businessman with extremely busy schedules. He was constantly on the move, ever coming up with one development project after the other. His business too kept evolving. It was impossible for him to stop for even one minute, he was always busy. Hardly had he completed a project than the next was ready to be launched. He was ever engaged on some activity, or attending a meeting somewhere. One day he was on a visit abroad, the next conquering a market somewhere else. Never a minute's pause to take a breather. His lifestyle was a constant flow of passionate and innovative activities.

He is now 87 years old and lives in an old people's home. He spends his time wandering along the corridors, tormented and with nothing anymore to keep him busy. It is an agonizing wait.... He feels depressed with no businesses to manage; his active life is in the past, and he cannot bear the situation. He feels lost and disoriented.

— Did I overwork myself too much and forgot to learn to be patient and nurture it…

The world today is constantly pushing us to always be busy doing something. Patience, however, is an open door towards simply being alive: a life of relaxation without anxieties.

| 3 |

| THE INSOMNIAC |

THE VIRTUES OF PATIENCE

"Sleep is the only friend
that does not respond when called".

Diane de Beausacq

— Doctor, I'm no longer able to go to sleep…., declares a young lady.

— Is that so? For how long has this been going on?

— It started a few months ago…. But for the last two weeks I've been able to fall asleep at best for two hours only.

The doctor looks at her and asks:

— Have you gone through some experience that might explain these bouts of insomnia?

— No, not really. I am naturally a stressed person with a very agitated lifestyle. For mc that's normal… I've not had any experience that has disrupted my lifestyle…

— Close your eyes. We are going to try and enact what happens when you sleep. Tell me what's going on in your mind…

— Umm… I'm thinking about my day tomorrow and what I'll need to do…. Then I tell myself: "Well, you need to sleep now".

— And then?

— And then, nothing…. I see the minutes, then the hours pass by.

— What do you tell yourself?

— The thoughts that come to my mind are: "Hey! I have to fall asleep!" she replied in exasperation.

— Fine. This is what you shall do tonight, said the doctor.

That evening the young lady stands in front of her bed and ponders:

— Alright. No medicine.... Just a sentence to repeat..... Given my situation, I think it would be best to follows the doctor's orders.

She lies on the bed and covers herself. She sets the alarm and starts, in a slow and low tone, to repeat to herself:

— I have decided to invite sleep.

Twenty minutes later, she was fast asleep with her fists clenched together.

It is easy to avoid falling into the trap of impatience by replacing attitudes of "I must" and "I should" in our lives by an attitude of good-will towards ourselves.

| 4 |

| THE SENTRY |

A NEW STATE OF MIND

"We often forget to stop and relish
the magic of the moment, whereas
that is what makes up basis of our lives".

Michel Bouthot

He was a sentry, keeping watch at the gate of a certain camp in the middle of the desert. All he saw in front of him every day was a large expanse of sand, thinly scattered with cactus plants, tough arborescent bushes and groves of yellowing grass. The hot, shiny yellow sun shone high in the sky above.

The sentry took up his post every morning at dawn, replacing the sentry who had been on guard at night.

You could say: "What a terrible life, having to withstand the same experience one day after the other".

You could say: "What a horrifying place this empty and dry desert is".

But the sentry never complained. He did not regret his destiny.

He had become wiser after having spent some time in the desert.

During his first year, he thought he would die out of boredom. He almost became depressed due to the quiet life and out of impatience.

The long wait almost had the better of him during the second year, and his whole body became agitated by the lack of activity.

By the fifth year he felt like an empty shell out of desperation.

However,….everything became clear to him during the sixth year: each day was different from the other. One day, the cacti blossomed, and the whole expanse burst with life, filling the day with a magic spell. Another time, the morning was calm and comforting, yet on another the day the sky was bright in full splendor… The desert was never the same again, perpetually hot and dry, with every day being the same. It was now filled with absolute peace.

Finally the sentry now had a different experience each day.

Life is made up of new experiences;

We need to relish them all.

| 5 |

| THE MUSICIANS |

SELF-CONFIDENCE

"Failure is first and foremost a feeling,
long before it becomes a reality.
It is the fruit of a combination of
vulnerability and a lack of self-confidence, that is thereafter
aggravated, usually deliberately, by fear".

Michelle Obama

Once upon a time there was a music conductor with exceptional talent. He was at the peak of his career, and all his fans had listened to his interpretations of the masterpieces by Bach, Mozart or Beethoven at least once. He was searching for four great violinists for his latest production. However, hardly any musician had the courage to come to his auditions, due to his strictness, high demands and talent. But a few mustered enough courage and appeared before him. Four remained after the rest had been eliminated, and they appeared before him. The first violinist played brilliantly, the second marvelously, the third splendidly, and the last impressively.

All the four sat in a small room, waiting for the master to make his choice. The *maestro* spent some time in his office, undecisive. He spent almost two hours going over the qualities of each violinist. In reality, he was impressed by the four musicians and was at a loss as to how to choose between them. He decided to inform them as follows: that he would employ them all. He opened his door and was surprised that there was only one violinist in the room!

— Where are the others? Asked the Master.

— The first one felt that your long hesitation was enough proof that he had not impressed you enough, so he left.

— And the second?

— He kept biting his nails, he was nervous… he could no longer wait and decided to go back home.

— And the third?

— When he saw the two other *virtuosos* give up and leave, he too felt he did not have any chance either.

— And what about you?

— Well, I guessed that the reason why you were taking so long must be that you liked the way we had played, and that I had an equal chance just like the rest, so I stayed.

Obviously, he is the one who got the job.

Your self-confidence
is the key to many opportunities.

| 6 |

| THE MILLIONNAIRE |

NO EFFORT, NO EXPECTATIONS

Do not waste your time
trying to please everybody.
Be the first priority in your life
and open your heart to happiness".

Rémi Ballot

The rich businessman is admiring all the possessions he has acquired at the peak of his life.

Beautiful paintings, vases set in precious stones, and furniture made from rare wood. In addition, he owns several yachts, apartments all over the world, as well as luxurious vehicles. Not forgetting fat bank accounts, he has everything you could ask for. He had worked hard to accumulate all this: he had sacrificed his whole life and energy for his personal success. However, the millionaire realized, lying on his deathbed, weakened and unable to move:

— So much hard work, sweat and stress to attain all this. So much energy spent to acquire all these objects. Now what more can I expect? There is nothing else to expect. Here I lie, surrounded by all these objects that I no longer need…

A voice whispered to him in a low tone:

— Perhaps you could start living all over, with no expectations and no desires whatsoever…

The man decided to try out the idea, and for the first time in his life, he felt at ease and at peace within himself, in a way that none of his businesses or his possessions had ever made him feel.

When we stop giving priority to
our possessions or achievements,
only one thing remains: life.
That is the magic of the simplicity of life.

| 7 |

| HIDDEN TREASURE |

ACTING WITH COMPASSION

"Desire is the price of
the success we dream of but are unable to attain,
wishes with no effect,
thoughts that are not realized".

Honoré de Balzac

He was convinced that this time around he had hit the jackpot! The explorer archeologist had for more than thirty years studied and carried out research on the Maya temple that had been lost and forgotten to mankind. Only he was aware of its existence.

He had dedicated his whole lifetime to it: a thesis and numerous visits to the place.... He was convinced that the monument was there, hidden somewhere between the mountains and the Amazon Forest. He also knew that a stone engraving would be found in this forgotten temple. According to Maya legend, the stone concealed the secret to priceless treasure.

Over and over again, he was convinced that finally he had found it. Despite his disappointments, he always resumed his search, each time more obsessed and determined than ever before.

To his relief, he finally succeeded in discovering the site of the temple. He was 70 years old then, but at last he had attained the objective of his lifetime, around which his whole existence revolved.

The temple is partially in ruins. The old man cautiously enters the main room. There is total silence all round, save for the man's heavy breathing and the chirping of birds in the nearby trees.

He walks towards a slab of stone: he is convinced that the valuable treasure is beneath it. He searches but finds nothing; except some writing. He blows away the dust and reads:

"*The only valuable treasure for mankind is to avoid being deluded by the mind*".

The writing hit him with a thud. It dawned on him that the obsession that had all along haunted his mind had ruined his entire life. Like an illusionary mental trap, it had prevented him from living a normal life.

It is possible to find the hidden inner treasure once you understand how the mind works, and free yourself from its control.

| 8 |

| THE PRESENT TIME AS IT IS |

ACCEPTANCE

"She relished the relaxed moments
of lethargy, planning nothing,
letting life go along uninterrupted,
and accepting everything as they came".

Delphine de Vigan

There was once upon a time a young hazelnut bush growing next to an imposing oak tree. It was summertime and the sunrays shot down magnificently from the clear sky.

— It's too hot! My roots can't reach the water, the hazelnut bush grumbled.

Soon autumn arrived, and with it came the rains, wind and cold temperatures. The two trees lost all their leaves.

— I feel naked without my leaves, what a horrible season! complained the hazelnut bush.

Come winter time, together with icy winds and frost. The ravens were flying low over the snow-laden fields, and kept cawing the entire day.

— My trunk will get messed up in all this brouhaha! Oh, what terrible weather this is! Mumbled the young bush. Springtime came, and our trees were soon covered in tender green leaves and budding flowers…

— What a pity that I am fast losing my beautiful flowers! Lamented the hazelnut bush. The oak tree, who had patiently remained silent the entire year, said to his young friend:

— Young plant, you have been complaining the whole year about what you are going through, or feeling bitterness for what was about to happen. Would you have rather died?

— No, not at all!

— Can you change the weather?

— No… unfortunately!

— Without a doubt. In such a case, the only thing you can change is yourself. Accept things as they are. Autumn will sprinkle you with water, winter will be a time for rest. Spring will wake you up while summer will make you fruitful. That's the way of life. You should accept and acknowledge it, since in reality there's nothing better you can do. Otherwise you'll never be happy. The young hazelnut bush could not agree more with the oak tree, as his only wish was to be happy. He thus decided to take life as it came.

It is impossible to bring everything in life under your control. Life is full of surprises and the unexpected. It is advisable to accept life as it is and to stop trying to dominate over everything.

| 9 |

| THE REED |

IMPARTIALITY

"The secret to a happy life used to be having a short memory".

Jojo Moyes

An old reed was growing on the ground. It seemed to have always been fixed on that spot. A young heron, feeling sorry for it, informed it:

— A storm is coming, and I'm flying away to escape it. Unfortunately for you, a stalk planted on the ground, you will be forced to endure winds strong enough to bring down an oak tree. You stand no chance at all…

— I've nothing to fear. Do you see this marshland? A hundred years ago it was all covered in trees. They all fell, tossed to the ground by strong winds and storms. I saw them, and I shall see more, I'm not afraid.

— What did you do? What's your secret? Asked the heron in surprise.

— My secret? I don't resist, I watch.

— I don't understand, remarked the bird.

— Well, I don't go against the winds whenever they blow on me. I just let them blow as much as they want as I watch.

— And?

— That's it, concluded the reed.

Like a reed that bends under the storm without breaking, are you able to allow your thoughts and life's events occur as you watch without interrupting?

| 10 |

| THE ALLURE OF A SMILE |

THE VIRTUES OF PATIENCE

"Laughter and sleep
are the best medicines in the world".

Irish Proverb

One Monday morning, under the grey Parisian sky, a young cashier – let us call her Alice – was on her way to work. As was the case every Monday, she did not feel like going to work. It was cold and rainy, yet it was just the first day of this week in the month of November. She realized that she was not the only one in a foul mood: everyone walked around with their faces looking as grumpy as a bulldog's. Passengers in the subway sat in silence, faces all gloomy and preoccupied.

She eventually reaches the office. She does not like her job. He boss barks the day's instructions in an authoritative tone.

The customers are standing in a queue as usual. The hall is crowded, the customers are cold and impolite. All look downcast and seem to be carrying the world's burdens on their shoulders.

For Alice, even as the day draws to a close, everything, like her life, appears gloomy. She begins to believe that she is worth nothing, that he is stuck in her lackluster lifestyle, and she feels lost.

A bubbly young woman rouses her suddenly from her dreamworld:

— Thanks for everything! See you soon! Remarked the woman as she finished arranging her shopping that Alice had tossed absentmindedly into the trolley.

— Umm.... You're welcome. Bye! Replied Alice with a tinge of discomfort.

The young woman gives her a big smile, just like that. It did not seem much, but Alice felt some positive vibration deep within her. The young woman had given her a little joy and some confidence within her.

What about you? How many people do you come across like this young woman every day?

| 11 |

| MEDITATION AT ANY COST |

THE VIRTUES OF PATIENCE

"Our best brains affirm
that this whole story is totally,
scientifically and realistically impossible.
But the story is not about being an impossibility,
it is only concerned about being realistic".

Pierre Pairault

— That's it! I'll start meditating from tomorrow! Charlotte, a nervous young woman, informed her friends.

Her enthusiasm was an expression of sheer determination. She embarks on the sessions the following day, but unfortunately she does not have the patience to continue for more than five minutes.

Her commitment fades as the days pass by. She always had one excuse or the other, each time there was something else that needed to be done: "I don't have the time tonight, I need to work on this file", "Oh, no! I shall do it tomorrow, I haven't done my shopping yet", or even, "I'm very tired tonight", or, "I'll go out instead for a drink in town, that will make me feel better".

However, at the end of every week, she makes a commitment to start all over, in vain.... There was always something more important that required her attention.... The years go by.... Upon her retirement, Charlotte is still searching without success for some exercise to take up.

She decides to seek advice from a diligent practicing meditator she knows, and who lives in the same neighborhood.

She got a very lucid answer:

— Any time you wish to embark on meditating, your mind will always divert your attention to something else.

— So, what can I do to overcome this challenge? Charlotte pleaded.

— It's not a question of what you should do, or desire, or have. All you need is just to be…

The first step towards patience and inner peace is just to be, consciously and deliberately, without paying attention to thoughts that divert us from our actions and desires.

| 12 |

| THE STRONGEST OF ALL ANIMALS |

A NEW MINDSET

"You become respectful when you get a bit of power,
but contemptuous when there is nothing
that you need from others.
You have faithfully followed the rule
that brought you to your current position:
Strong among the weak, and weak among the strong".

Karine Tuil

As is usually the behavior among animals, there were always brawls to decide who was the strongest, the bravest or the most powerful. *Egos* confronted one another in long noisy exchanges, howling, cackles, and at times the differences were settled through paw and tooth fights.

The tiger was on that day explaining to the rest of the animals how he was the strongest of all. The big elephant sneered at this, and seizing a huge mango tree with his trump, uprooted it completely off the ground. Everybody agreed that the elephant was the strongest of all animals. The pachyderm strutted around with pride, very pleased with himself.

But the tiger stepped in to ask him:

— Tell me, Elephant, how much do you weigh?

— I weigh six tons!

— And how much weight can you lift?

— Humans say that I can lift nine tons.

All the other animals cried out in amazement…

But the tiger, licking his fur, said:

— Quite impressive… As for me, I can lift more than five hundred kilos! That is twice my weight! Proportionally, I'm thus stronger than you.

All the animals became quiet in their admiration, and came to the tiger to congratulate him.

But perched on a rock, a meek dung beetle, cried out:

— All that's very good... but what about me?

The tiger, the elephant and all the other animals burst out in laughter:

— You can't be serious! Who would admire you? You spend your time pushing a ball of dung all over the plain! Is that what you call… your strength?

— Dear friends, I'd like to remind you that we dung beetles are useful for cleaning your waste, and therefore you should acknowledge our importance…

The tiger and the elephant exchanged uneasy glances, but did not utter a word.

— … our strength, continued the dung beetle, if we are to follow tiger's calculations, is way above yours in measure: indeed, every day, in my modest way, I push, pull and carry more than… a thousand times my weight.

From that day, all the animals, ill at ease, ended their constant disputes and departed, each their own way, to meditate over this small lesson on humility.

There is no doubt that we all have our own inner strengths and resources. Our self-esteem comes alive perhaps only after we become aware of this.

| 13 |

| THE ROMAN FIGHTER |

SELF-ESTEEM

"Do you have to grow old
in order to appreciate the passage of time,
go on a strict diet for a week
to appreciate a good meal,
deny yourself so as to deserve pleasure?"

Michel Bussi

Once upon a time, in ancient Rome, there lived a young gladiator named Nimrod.

All manner of men, fighters and soldiers always lost their fights against him. However determined or aggressive they were (please note that none of them were mere choirboys), on the day of combat, they all entered into the arena trembling with fear, fought clumsily before biting the dust in front of the mysterious fighter. Young Nimrod, noting that there were no other opponents to quench his thirst for more victory and honors, decided to challenge an old fighter who was busy sharpening his sword in the open, right next to the arena. The old man mumbled some words, hesitated, deep in thought, then finally accepted the challenge.

I should at this point reveal to you Nimrod's secret of success: He had in his youth acquired a little demon, who used to fly out at night to whisper into the left ear of his master's challengers all sorts of deceptive messages. By morning they would be demoralized, and with no more fighting spirit in them, they would be easily defeated. On the eve of the fight, Nimrod sent the demon to go and discourage the old man by whispering negative words in his left ear as he slept. In the morning, Nimrod entered the arena already smelling success as he was accustomed to. He, however, became rather uneasy when he noticed the old man coming in calmly, with no sign of fear on his face. Once the combat began, he realized that his challenger was quite determined to win! Nimrod started wondering what was going on. He hesitated, breathing heavily, and in no time the old fighter beat him to the ground.

Nimrod, lying on the ground, with his mouth full of blood, asked the old man:

— Old man… tell me, how have you managed to defeat me?

— Huh? Can you speak a bit louder? said the old fighter. I can't hear you, I'm deaf on my left ear!

Others might try to impose themselves over you sometimes. Your best defenses are your confidence and composure.

| 14 |

| HE WHO WISHED TO BECOME AN INSTRUCTOR |

NO EFFORT, NO EXPECTATIONS

"The further away we are from an occurrence, the more difficult it is for us to identify its possible cause".

Russell Banks

An experienced meditation instructor had achieved a lot of success. His classes were always full and he got more and more students. One day, one of his followers, an impatient and spirited young man, who had consistently studied meditation for several years, asked:

— Can you tell me how long it will take for me to become an accomplished meditation instructor? He was full of enthusiasm and pride.

The instructor mulled over the question for a moment, then replied coldly:

— The way I see it, thirty years.

The student replied, very uneasy and disappointed:

— Well, ... that's quite a long time! What if I worked on it without a rest, if I thought about it day and night, if I trained intensively in meditation, if I practiced without slackening? How long will it take me?

At this the instructor was once again deep in thought for a longer time, then replied:

— In such a case I would say fifty years.

— What! exclaimed the student… So, what should I do? Please tell me, I'm ready to do whatever it takes!

— Every effort that you make takes you further away from the real principles of meditation.

Meditation is not a competition where relentlessness and hard work are the in-things to do… It is a question of just being there. Nothing more.

| 15 |

| COLORS OF LIFE |

ACTING WITH COMPASSION

"Sight is probably
always influenced by something,
and depends on the ability
to compare one thing
from the other".

Vidiadhar Surajprasad Naipaul

This is the story of twin brothers. They are similar in all physical characteristics, but have totally different personalities: one views everything from a negative angle, always suspicious to the extreme, even to the point of despising himself; the other is an optimist by nature, self-confident, appreciating himself and others. Apart from their similar physical characteristics, they dress the same, walk in the same manner, though they have different temperaments.

As a result of this "love-hate" relationship between the two, they became the subjects of numerous studies by experts who tried to find out how twins brought up under virtually identical circumstances could have such different characters.

Their lives had followed virtually the same path. They attended the same schools, and took up similar professions. Indeed, they lived parallel lives.

One twin, however, was disappointed with his life and was miserable. His brother, on the other hand, was satisfied: he lived a moderate and happy life.

Whereas it is in reality possible to compare lifestyles, one factor can considerably change how we take it: our inner mindset.

If you view your days with a dark mindset, your life will be likewise; if you color them brightly, your life will also be more luminous.

| 16 |

| PATIENCE AND ACCEPTANCE |

ACCEPTANCE

"Your friend is the solution to all your needs.
He is the garden that you sow with love
and harvest with thanksgiving.
He is your table filled with food and he gives warmth.
You come to him when you are hungry
and look for him when you want peace".

Khalil Gibran

It happened a very long time ago. Astrologers from two neighboring kingdoms were categorical: The harvests were going to be poor: ravaging insects in very large numbers as well as a looming famine were going to affect the land in the coming years. The two kings believed their astrologers even though their predictions were particularly worrying. The first king decided to do something about it: he had the fields tilled twice instead of once, and had them irrigated more than usual. The farmers were instructed to put manure on their farms to improve their fertility, to weed and work tirelessly. When the insects arrived, the farmers spent entire nights collecting them by hand and destroying them. Despite their relentless efforts, for several years the harvest remained poor. The people were filled with worry and fatigue, but their hearts were still filled with reverence for their king. They could all imagine how the situation would have been had he not taken any steps at all. In the other kingdom, however, the king had encouraged everyone… to remain patient. He advised all to save their strength and not to damage the soil.

The farmers did not till the land, but planted their crops among the weeds and other adventitious plants. They did not water the crops much, and the only crops that grew were the more resistant ones that did not need a lot of water. They did not bother with the insects, and whereas the first year was difficult, the abundance of locusts and green flies attracted such a large number of predators that the farmers did not need to take any action. Furthermore, the weeds were enough food for other animals that would otherwise have eaten the crops. The kingdom was thus able to withstand with ease the crisis that had been announced, and everyone was thankful for their king's wisdom.

We encounter in life times that are more difficult than others, some gloomy days more than others. Patience is a virtue that enables us to affirm that all is just temporary: it is wiser to wait in confidence that change will come.

| 17 |

| THE GOSSIPERS |

IMPARTIALITY

"If you are distressed over something,
that is not what is troubling you,
it is rather your judgement of it".

Marc Aurèle

Two female friends liked to meet often at café terraces to engage on their favorite topic: gossip.

— Look at the dress that lady is wearing!

— My God! She should be told about it. And have you seen that other one, over there? She is smart and has beautiful hair, but her walking style.... Reminds me of a penguin..

— Oh, and that one, over there, near the waiter. What a horrible neck-line.

— And the waiter, he looks really common-class.

— That's why he is a waiter! And look at the guy near the entrance...

— He's totally stuck in time.... Just look at his coat! My Gosh! You'd think we're still living in the 1980's!

They spent hours on end laughing, judging, mocking and analyzing everybody around. They did this for several years.

One day, however:

— Just see how that lady is carrying herself around, thinking that she is beautiful. She imagines she is Miss World.

— You should stop thinking that you could be Miss Universe when you are no longer young. And the way she is showing off!

A man was sitting just behind the two gossipers. He was unable to concentrate on his newspaper due to their endless chatter. He finally decided to leave, but before doing so, he removed a small mirror from his bag

He came to the table where the two sat and briefly placed the mirror in front of each of their faces.

— Have a nice day, he said as he walked towards the exit.

Who judges us when we judge others? Do we consider ourselves to be perfect or superior as we judge others?

| 18 |

| THE MASTER AND THE SAMURAI |

THE VIRTUES OF PATIENCE

"It is impossible to understand mankind,
they believe that they have
a new life waiting for them elsewhere.
They are always dreaming of a lost paradise".

Dominique Blondeau

A Japanese Zen tale recounts the story of a Samurai who went before Hakuin, the Zen master and asked him:

— Do heaven and hell really exist?

— Who are you? asked the master as he rested in the garden surrounded by trees gently swaying in the wind.

— I am Tomoshi, a Samurai, he replied haughtily and with disdain, as the man did not seem to have recognized his fame.

— You, a warrior! exclaimed Hakuin. Don't make me laugh! Which master would want you to serve him? You are dressed like a beggar.

Filled with great anger, the Samurai reached for his sword, ready to strike.

Hakuin continued:

— At least you have a sword! But you're too clumsy to cut off my head! You're not worthy to be carrying it.

The Samurai, filled with rage, lifted his sword, ready to strike the master, who calmly replied:

— That's the opening of the door to hell.

The Samurai was taken aback by the monk's relaxed countenance. He put back his sword and bowed before him.

— That's where the door to heaven opens, remarked the master.

The beginning of wisdom is when we become aware of the total power of our minds. The beginning of patience is when we start to slowly take control.

| 19 |

| NOISES |

THE VIRTUES OF PATIENCE

"The only things
that increase today
are noise levels".

Georges Picard

The drummer of a famous rock group was forced to interrupt his tour when the doctor informed him of the cause of his illness. The diagnosis hit him with a thud: tinnitus.

He had to be replaced. But for him the worst was yet to come: his mind was overrun by all kinds of unbearable noises that cut him off from the outside world and gave him constant headaches.

He became irritable, and grew increasingly impatient, nervous, always on edge: He felt sick all the time and his tinnitus worsened. His whole life revolved around his condition and his moments of anguish. The noises in his mind became more and more unbearable. Our musician's life turned to one of anguish, with the future outlook being a permanent fear of crisis after crisis.

The mere sight of a musical instrument made him want to throw up. He became depressed, lonely and embittered.

One day he stumbled upon a book on wisdom. One sentence captured his attention: "Only the present is real: concentrate your mind on the moment". He instantly became aware of his expectations, and he realized what his life had become: tinnitus had become to him an obsession that was poisoning his life.

— Now is the time to make a change, he resolved.

He conditioned himself to always think only of the moment. Oh! His illness did not go away, however… But it now became just one of life's problems, and did not stop him from engaging in other things, in going about his life in the present. He even managed to form a new musical group.

You live life in the present. You do not gain anything by worrying about the future before it comes. You will just suffer in vain.

| 20 |

| THE ACTOR AND THE BEGGAR |

A NEW MINDSET

"After all, what do we gain by always looking back to our past and blaming ourselves when our lives do not take the path exactly as we would have wished?"

Kazuo Ishiguro

The famous actor's career had been a life of one success after the other. Full concerts filled with applause exhilarated him night after night. He was praised, celebrated, admired. His voice recited pieces by best-selling authors. His acting had brought to life works by Shakespeare, Musset, Racine... He became filled with pride, but as he was aware that this would send away his admirers, he play-acted his real life as a "modest" person. One day, he came across a beggar who asked him for alms. With an air of condescendence, he held out a ten Euro bill to him, at the same time advising him to look for a job.

— And, sir, where would you want me to look for a job?

— I don't know,... anywhere?

— Do you think that life is that simple in my situation?

— I know a little about your kind of life, I've played the part of a beggar in a few plays, replied the actor.

— Was any of them about me? Asked the beggar, feigning surprise.

— Umm, no... but it was the part of a beggar, so...

— ...Oh, is that so? In that case, are all people who give alms the same?

— Umm... I didn't say that.... But there are similarities.

— Let's be frank with each other: am I in the streets through my own fault or by bad luck?

— A bit of both.

— So, in a way I deserve my fate?

— Obviously you're responsible for it in a way, replied the actor, getting increasingly embarrassed.

— Does it not bother you, saying such things about me while you know nothing at all? The actor turned and walked away, glad that no one had heard what had gone on. He decided to concentrate on his *a priori*.

It is never wise to blame anyone under distress. One of life's most important rules is to remain humble even when good fortune blows your way.

| 21 |

| THE SEEDS |

SELF-CONFIDENCE

"Keeping your humility in all,
remaining respectful in your beliefs".

Hugh Laurie

An aged farmer, at the point of his death, could feel the heavy burden of his many years. All his life he had been a good, just and hard-working man. He had four sons and was at pains to choose who among them would take over his small farm. He decided to leave everything to the most honest of them.

He summoned all his sons to his bedroom and told them:

— My sons, I'm growing weaker every day and soon I'll no longer be with you. I need to choose one of you to cultivate my fields and keep the farm beautiful and prosperous. I've therefore decided to give each one of you a seed. After four weeks, whoever will have put his seed to the best use will have proved to be the best one to inherit the farm.

The four boys left the room and each went on his way to plant his precious seed. One of them planted his in a pot, another in a compost heap. A third planted his on plain ground, while the last planted his on a heath-mound... The youngest son was called Basile, and as much as he tried, watering, warming and placing his pot in the sunshine… the seed did not germinate. He however did not want to cheat, as that would be a shameful act. He thus worked on bravely, refusing to be overcome by despair, but with no success! Two weeks later, the father called all his sons to come with their pots. Three of the sons walked in, each proudly carrying their pot with a beautiful plant growing in it. Basile, however, walked in with an empty pot and his eyes full of tears… He had to accept that his other brothers were better than him. The father turned towards him and said:

— Well, my son, the farm goes to you.

The other three brothers protested vigorously, pointing out that nothing was growing in their youngest brother's pot.

— Precisely, replied the father. Those old seeds were useless, they had taken in too much water last year… If yours grew, that's proof that you threw away the seed I'd given you and replaced it with another! There's no doubt therefore that the one who took the best care of the seed I had given is Basile, and not any of you others!

Basile was happy to have stayed true to himself.

Being honest and consistent with yourself is the best way to live your life and to develop a reliable personality.

| 22 |

| AWARENESS |

NO EFFORT, NO EXPECTATIONS

"It is a good thing to have faith in the past: the future will always open to us its secrets".

Eve Belisle

Inside the building of a large multinational company. Three men dressed in impeccable suits are waiting patiently outside the office of the Human Resources Director. They are waiting for a job interview for an opening in senior management.

Two of them are nervous: they are restless, pacing up and down. As for the third, he was calm and sat in silence.

— How come you are able to stay so calm? Asked one of the other two in a stressed tone.

— I'm impressed, said the other. As for me, I'm in such a panic.

— You too? Asked the first. That's a relief… I'm always scared of making a blunder.

— As for me, I'm not equal to the task, the second confirmed. You on the other hand are so relaxed one would think you were in a doctor's waiting room…

— Well... I'm not really sure. Let's just say that I don't have special qualities or better qualifications than any of you. But I'm aware of whatever I possess.

The door opened at that moment and the director asked our man to go in. He stood up and walked with confidence towards the office.

The other two candidates looked at each other in surprise. They even thought of leaving before sitting for the interview, as the confidence of the man had left such an impression on them.

Self-awareness is an important leverage for personal confidence and esteem. This is a reminder to the popular Greek saying: "know yourself".

| 23 |

| COMPARING IS NOT REASONING |

ACTING CONSCIOUSLY

"It is only after
thoroughly comparing the facts
that the wisest man will
appreciate the difference between them".

Mary Ann Evans

The plant in the under-bush was engrossed in thought:

— My friends, she said to the thorn-bushes beside her. Do you see how different I am from you all? I don't have any thorns to defend myself, I'm not as big as you are either. I'm not like anything else, I'm just ugly.

The following day she talked to the shrubs:

— See how different I am from you, my friends. I'm not as majestic as you are, nor do I have beautiful branches. In comparison I'm just tiny and shriveled. You on the other hand are huge and look impressive.

It was obvious that this plant was not happy. She was the only one of her species in the area.

She called out to a squirrel that passed by her every day:

— You are so lucky to have such beautiful fur, and also to be able to move around. As for me, I don't have any of that.

As the sunrays pierced through the overgrowth, the squirrel could not help but remind her.

— You are the most beautiful of all the plants and animals. Even as you compare yourself to others, haven't you noticed your colored petals that illuminate the under-bush? Are you not aware of your perfume that smalls so beautiful?

Indeed, the plant had mutated into a magnificent wild flower with a such a refined perfume that everyone admired.

Comparing is not the same as reasoning: the silent voice in us is always inclined to making us see what we do not have instead of our true worth.

| 24 |

| ACCEPTANCE IS NOT SUBMISSION |

ACCEPTANCE

"We talk of freedom all the time
in European cultures.
However, for most of us
this freedom does not refer to the freedom to choose
from the several possibilities that nature provides, rather, it
is a submission
to our wishes and desires".

Bernard Minier

A mercenary found himself caught in a snowstorm, and sought refuge in a cave. It was cool and fresh in there, and the sweet smell of incense filled the air: for several years, a hermit had lived in the cave, and he was reputed to be very wise.

The soldier met him and asked for a meal. The hermit gladly shared with him his gruel.

— What! Is this all you eat? Food fit only for swine? I only eat the finest foods given to me by my partners!

— As for me, I eat whatever I can get, and I usually find it very delicious. I accept whatever comes my way: the wind, the rain, the cold, as well as fruits and visitors…

— Ugh! I can't understand how you can bear just being there, with no life, waiting like a fool instead of…

— Yes? Instead of what?

— Taking control of your life! Setting the pace of your life! Shouted the mercenary.

— I do set the pace of my life! I decide where I want to be, like now, to be here. I meditate every day and so I am consciously in control of every second in my life. I lead my life as I wish!

— So, you take life as it comes, huh? You're such a milksop!

The wise man gave the soldier a loud smack…. who, after a moment of confused surprise, drew out his sword and shouted:

— I'm going to kill you!

— Perhaps…. But as you can see, I live my life as I wish, I'm freer than you are, I'm not scared of dying, and I don't like it when I offer someone a meal and they decide to insult me instead… As for everything else, let whatever must happen, happen…

And without paying further attention to the shining blade extended towards him, the wise man turned to his meal while smiling broadly to the fighter.

The mercenary could not help but admire the power of his host's character. He sat down, lost in thought.

Acceptance is not a sign of submission or weakness: on the contrary, it means being true to your personal choices.

| 25 |

| A FAMILY STORY |

IMPARTIALITY

"Never judge others.
You do not know
what is distressing them
deep in their hearts".

Mary Higgins Clark

A villager did not want to take the main route going to town. He decided to take a longer route that took an hour more. Why? Well, the main route passed through another village where a family they had quarreled with generations ago lived. His great-grandfather, his grandfather and his father had all advised him never to go to the "accursed village", where the nearest farm belonged to their rival family. Ever since he was a young child, he always looked from afar at the house with contempt whenever he was going to town. On that fateful day, however, his vehicle broke down.

The weather was stormy and wet. Night was falling on the moorland and the rain was falling so hard he could hardly breath. His only option was to walk. He hesitated when he reached the crossroads. He had the choice of taking the route that skirted round the accursed village (which meant walking for a further two hours), or go and seek help from the village.

— I can't lower my dignity and ask them for help. These are bad people, full of hatred and my fore-fathers had always told me that they are ever looking forward to our ruin…

He got caught up in a strong gust of wind and he fell down. He had no choice. He entered the village and knocked on the door of the family to ask for help. He was expecting them to release their dogs on him or insult him, indeed, make jibes at him.

He was very surprised to realize that instead he was warmly received. He was offered a meal and given a towel to dry himself. He was asked to stay until the storm went down. Our villager was somewhat embarrassed as he was leaving the following morning…

— And I thought that we really hated each other… They were not even aware of our old quarrels. They were so polite to me.

We sometimes become prisoners of our own prejudices and past histories.

Aren't they rather obstacles in our lives?

26 |

| PATIENCE OF A GENERAL |

THE VIRTUES OF PATIENCE

"I have always admired the look on the face of a person
who has lost, their eyes,
the yawns, the doubts, silence, all say a lot.
Victory makes a fool of you.
Defeat brings about fascinating hiatus.

Nicolas Delesalle

A strategist of the Athenian army was considering trying out a new plan for defeating their Spartan enemies. He decided to consult the oracle at Pythia, in the temple of Delphia. Speaking from the dark inner part of the temple, the oracle said: "Victory will be yours when the ground under your feet becomes wet".

"What a strange prophecy", he said to himself.

One week later, the Spartan army advanced dangerously close. The generals moved forward to meet them, in accordance with the advice from Pythia. The rain suddenly began to fall. "The soil is getting wet! Here's the fulfilment of the prophecy!" said his assistant.

But it was not the right moment yet for the strategist. Nobody else around him understood. Some of his commanders thought that something had gone wrong with him, for his passivity was unusual. They thus gave the order to attack without waiting for instructions from their commander.

They came back the following morning feeling remorseful. The attack had failed. Worse still, they had to inform the strategist of the death of his son, who had been one of the soldiers involved.

He could not hold back his tears. He fell to his knees and wept. He wept for a long time, but soon noticed that the ground around him had become soaked in his tears.

He leapt up on his feet.

— Let's go, victory is ours!

The Athenians pushed back the Spartans completely. The strategist was highly acclaimed for his wisdom and patience in war.

As was the case with this general, patience always pays if you wait for the right moment.

| 27 |

| LOCKED UP INDOORS |

THE VIRTUES OF PATIENCE

"You need to wait for nightfall to be able to see the stars, and it is also strange that in all great investigations, the detectives always have to wait for the dark so as to be able to start seeing any light".

Arthur Upfield

It was the beginning of spring, and two marmots were waking up from their hibernation. They stretched themselves in the burrow they had slept in.

— I have such a mammoth hunger!

— Me too. After sleeping through the winter season, I need to look for something to eat. .

One of the marmots stuck out its snout at the opening of the burrow. The clean mountain air was very refreshing.

She rushed back into the safety of the burrow upon seeing a hungry fox in the distance looking for prey.

— What's the matter? Asked the friend.

— We need to wait a bit longer before going to look for something to eat. There's a fox out there looking for prey.

— Sorry, I'm too hungry. I can't wait any longer in this hole.

— You must be crazy! Have a little patience until the fox goes away.

— No way! I've come across foxes thousands of times in my life, he won't be able to catch me..

She discreetly leaves the burrow and starts to browse on the grass. After around ten minutes, she calls out to her friend:

— Come on over! There's nothing to fear, you were worried over nothing..

But the fox had crept in from behind, pounced on the marmot and held her firmly in his jaws.

Learning to wait

and controlling the desires

of the body and mind

is the secret to wisdom.

| 28 |

| THE PEASANTS |

A NEW MINDSET

"Life is a big game,
you draw your cards,
choose the best,
and hold on to the trump cards".

Agnès Ledig

It was a very long time ago. Two peasants, one young and other older, were working hard sowing large farms. The radiant sun high up in the sky was a sign of a hot day ahead.

The young peasant kept complaining while the older one worked on. They tossed armfuls of wheat all over the freshly tilled land.

— Old man, for how long have you been doing this work?

— Slightly over thirty years.

— How tiresome, don't you find these farms too large?

The older peasant smiled and said:

— It's because you're not using enough strength and precision in your arms. See how I do it.

He took a handful of wheat and, with a skillful twist of his hand, scattered the seeds far and wide. The younger farmer, with a tinge of envy, replied:

— Is that it? See me do it also.

With that he tossed a handful of seeds.

— Not bad, responded the old man. But I'm sure I can do better than you in the farm.

— Deal! Said the young man, infuriated.

The two set out to sow another farm in total concentration, and as quickly as each of them could.

— I'm beating you! The old man said.

— You're not even an inch ahead of me! Responded the younger farmer.

When they finished sowing the farm, the old farmer came to the younger man:

— So, tell me, was this work as tiresome as with the other farms?

— Of course not! We had a bet on this one.

— There was no bet, it was just a game, replied the old man. I want you to learn that it's possible to take things seriously and work hard, but at the same time have the mindset of a child: What I mean is, you can take pleasure in anything that you do, so long as you consider it as a game.

Life is a game:

Everything becomes easier

once you take it that way.

| 29 |

| AUTOMATIC GEAR |

SELF-CONFIDENCE

"To be able to do great things,
you need a measure of insensitivity,
to leave out the smaller ones
that cling on you wherever you go.
Unless you come across a small one
that grows and becomes great".

Charles Messager

There was once a bizarre-looking bridge over a certain mountain: it was a long rope attached to two ends over a valley, and only those who were daring enough had the courage to use it. There was a sign on one end of the rope that read: "Be Light Without Being Crazy"..

Three men, all out of breath, arrived at the foot of the bridge. They were messengers from the king and they had an urgent letter to deliver. They had decided to take this shortcut in order to save time.

They hesitated when they saw the bridge, and the gaping valley below.

The first messenger, his entire body trembling in fear, decided to cross the bridge. As he advanced, he kept thinking: "I'm going to fall, I'm going to fall....

There's no doubt about it, I'm going to fall..." Sure enough, he fell halfway across the bridge.

The second messenger stepped on the bridge, his whole body shaking in fear too. His face was red with fear. As he crossed, he thought: "It's so easy! There's absolutely no danger! I shouldn't worry at all..." But he too, fell halfway across the bridge.

The third messenger, trembling even more than the other two, stepped on the bridge. He had seen his two friends perish in the valley below. His heart beat so loudly he thought it would fall out of his chest.

He said to himself: "Be still, dear heart. This is a test that we shall go through together. Be still, dear body. This is a test that we shall go through together. Be strong, dear mind. This is a test that we shall go through together". He reached the other end of the bridge as he kept repeating this, though he was hardly able to contain his courage. He resumed his running to continue with his mission.

Every step you take towards your goal

is a sure sign of victory.

| 30 |

| EXPECTATIONS (OF THE MIND) |

NO EFFORT, NO EXPECTATATIONS

"The success of a great cause
is not measured solely
by attaining its final objective.
You are already victorious if you can
rise above your expectations in your lifetime".

Nelson Mandela

One day, a farmer received a beautiful white horse as a present for his son. It was a magnificent animal and everyone in the village admired it.

The following day, one of his neighbors came to admire the horse and to congratulate the farmer:

— You are so lucky! I don't expect to ever receive such a beautiful white horse as a gift!

To which the farmer replied:

— I'm not sure if it's a good or bad thing.

A few weeks later, the farmer's son tried to ride the horse, which seemed to be rather restive; it sent him flying into the air. The young man broke his leg, and for a very long time, he was unable to help his parents around the farm.

— Oh, how unfortunate! Exclaimed the neighbor. You were right to say this could have been a bad thing. Now your son is disabled. How are you going to ensure all the harvesting is completed without his helping hand?

The farmer responded:

— I'm not sure if it's a good or bad thing.

Several weeks passed by after the accident. The war had broken out: all young men in the village were called to register. The farmer's son, however, was not conscripted due to his broken leg.

The neighbor came back to him and said:

— All the young men of the village, except your son, have been conscripted into the war; he surely is so lucky!

The farmer repeated his usual remark:

— I'm not sure if it's a good or bad thing.

Life continues regardless of what happens. If we impose our expectations to it, we run the risk meeting disappointment and misfortune.

| 31 |

| TRANSFORMATION |

ACTING CONSCIOUSLY

"The main characteristic of unselfish kindness
is being unrecognized,
unknown, invisible, and above suspicion
– a good act that shouts out
is never unselfish".

Amélie Nothomb

There once lived a crooked man. He had lived a life of theft and lies. He was a manipulating and cruel man, always angry at everything and everybody. He stopped at nothing in his way of life.

One day he was taking a stroll when he came face to face with a hermit. He was highly impressed by the wise man's composure, and before he realized it, he had fallen on his knees, beseeching him to enlighten him and to help him find forgiveness for his evil lifestyle.

The old mand smiled at him and pointed out to him an old tree that had been struck and charred by lightning:

— Do you see that dead old tree? Well, you shall be forgiven when it blossoms once again!

In disappointment, the man flew into a furious rage:

— You might as well have said that I'll never be forgiven, retorted the man. In that case, I should just continue with my usual lifestyle.

The man went on his way, and continued with his wayward life, tormenting everyone he came across.

One day as he walked towards an old farm, he saw through the window a woman and her hungry children. They were sitting around a pot, and she was singing to them a lullaby: “Go to sleep, my children. Mummy’s preparing food. Go to sleep, sleep till morning”.

Intrigued, he waited till the woman left the room. He tiptoed into the room and lifted the pot’s lid: it was filled with stones. The man shrugged his shoulders and removed the stones from the pot. He took from his bag a piece of mutton that he had stolen from elsewhere, cut it into pieces and threw them into the pot. He relit the fire under the pot before going on his way. He was extremely touched by the sheer misery and misfortune of the sad family.

That day, the old tree blossomed once again.

What changed our man was the unselfish act: he received forgiveness when he opened up his heart.

| 32 |

| THE PRISONERS |

ACCEPTANCE

"Meditation is self-effacement,
it means silence and openness,
acceptance with no conflict of interests".

Arnaud Desjardins

A very long time ago, two men were imprisoned after having been wrongly convicted. They were tied with strong ropes and left in a yard awaiting their execution.

A philosopher contemplating the situation would have concluded that the ropes symbolized a man's thoughts unconsciously coiling around his mind. Even when you do not want to think anymore, the line is always there to tie in the mind.

The first man was forceful and prone to violence. He was used to being in charge, to be the head, and boasted of living his life like a ship's captain. He was furious at being accused falsely. He pulled at the rope, fought and struggled with all his strength.

The second man, on the other hand, was more composed. He accepted life as it came, the blows from fate and the instability of our possessions. He knew and accepted that injustice was a reality. He could do nothing against it, and twisting or contracting his body would not help either.

The first man shouted at him: “Coward! Move, do something! Are you just going to endure and do nothing, you weakling?”.

However, the other man did not say anything. He breathed in quietly and relaxed his whole body. After a short while, his body became so supple and flexible that he could easily untie the rope that held him down. He freed his friend and they both managed to escape without much problem.

It does not serve any purpose to harden your heart against life. Accept things as they come, for, as is the case in this story, it is not a matter of doing nothing or leaving things as they are.

| 33 |

| SELF-LOVE |

IMPARTIALITY

"Most people
desire more to be admired than to be loved.
Admiration satisfies the ego,
that exists in all people.
Friendship is a feeling,
that many people do not possess".

Marie-Geneviève-Charlotte Darlus, (1760)

A delegate in a conference completed his speech. He is a well-known personality, wealthy, admired and…. is living with a disability. He has lived his entire life in a wheelchair, as his body became deformed after a difficult birth.

However, he is full of life, and is admired by all. Someone from the audience timidly raises a slender hand. A frail young woman begins to speak. She too is in a wheelchair and only knows too well the challenges of living with disability:

— What can one do to succeed in life when you do not have the same chances as other people? You, like me, have not had the same chances since birth as everyone else…. but you have made it. I, on the other hand, have never managed to achieve anything… What's your secret?

The delegate smiled and replied as follows:

— I've always loved myself. If you love yourself, if you love your body with its capabilities and resources, your mind will cease to focus on the limitations. You will stop thinking about what you cannot do, and focus on what you can do.

We are all prone to lowering our worth and comparing ourselves. In this way, we limit the number of opportunities open to us.

| 34 |

| THE SHRUB WHO WISHED TO BE AN OAK TREE |

THE VIRTUES OF PATIENCE

"Happiness is this state of mind that enables you to love the present".

Patrick Bauwen

Two shrubs in a clearing are having a conversation:

— When I grow up, I'll be an oak tree. I shall be the tallest oak tree around. Oh, yes! That's for sure! He affirmed with a lot of conviction.

The second shrub just listened in good faith.

The same old story went on and on for several years:

— You'll see. My shadow will cover the whole of this area. You'll see! You'll all see, he added, addressing the other plants around. I'll be so tall that I'll protect all of you.

All the animals just smiled.

Years passed by. The shrub that had wished to become a tall oak tree kept on talking so much about the future that he forgot to produce enough sap. The other, on its part, while listening politely to the first shrub, ensured that it had produced sufficient sap to enable it grow into a majestic tree with beautiful leaves. It covered its friend who, still slender and fragile, had not even noticed that it was still so tiny. The little tree full of goodwill was well loved by all; he had a likeable personality.

But it never became the tall oak tree that it had so wished to be, far from it.

The strength of the present moment lies in the ability to always mobilize your skills for the future, and not the other way round.

| 35 |

| A NUMBER OF DAYS |

THE VIRTUES OF PATIENCE

"I learnt that patience
was the greatest,
most noble but most ignored virtue.
It has helped us to love the world
first before trying to transform it".

Sylvain Tesson

It was the Karate fighter's big day. He had been a diligent student who had practiced hard under the watchful eye of his trainer. He was expecting to be appointed as an instructor and thus achieve his dream of starting his own school and training others what he had learnt. He had been waiting for this for a long time and was a little impatient. He had prepared all that was needed: the equipment, the fees to be charged, the place, the exercises… everything.

However, luck was not on his side: a storm had broken out. It rained heavily for several days without stopping. The budding instructor paced up and down every morning, cursing at the storm which did not seem to be weakening.

He began to have doubts and to wonder; he decided to consult his trainer:

— Master, I'm very angry right now: I've worked so hard to become an instructor, and this storm is stopping me from going ahead to achieve my dreams.

The master did not reply.

— Master, what should I do?

— My friend, there's nothing you can do. You have worked hard training for many years, and have been patient all along. Can't you wait for just a few more days? Good weather always comes after the rains. Didn't I teach you about patience?

The student bowed at the master. He had understood that the greatest treasure in his training was not the physical skills acquired, but rather, patience and commitment.

| 36 |

| A CHILDLIKE SPIRIT |

A NEW MINDSET

"Children play games searching for treasure,
while adults search for honors.
There will never be an end to this".

Denis Tillinac

A certain gentleman had travelled a lot and filled up several passports. He had seen so much that nothing amazed him anymore. He became bored with the 5-Star hotels, the velvet covers, the starched furnishings. Nothing excited him any longer. He found himself trapped in France by the lockdowns, and he resigned himself to visiting his daughter and grandson. Our gentleman did not like his family much. His eight-year-old grandson did not really care about the expensive watch that our gentleman had bought for him as a gift. He was more interested in having his grandfather spend the night with him in the tree house he had built in the garden.

— Grandpa will love that, said his mother. He is an adventurer.

— Of course, said the grandfather, visibly piqued. I went on several safaris in Africa a few years ago.

The boy jumped up with excitement. He ran to fetch sleeping bags, as well as two torches, and made the beds. At bed-time the grandfather did not show any excitement at the thought of spending the night in the garden, virtually in the open sky.

— Just wait and see, it'll be a super-exciting adventure, said the grandson.

— You think so?

— Of course! Have you done this before?

— Umm… No…

— So, it'll be an adventure.

The old man lay down beside his grandson. He was amused by the boy's innocence, his surprise and excitement at playing with the dynamo-powered torch. His thoughts wandered to his own childhood. He remembered how everything impressed him then, how bread tasted so good… his own grandma's garden seemed so large… and how owning a chrome bicycle was such a wonderful dream. In an instant, our gentlemen, or rather, grandpa, reliving his childhood, could once more smell the grass, the freshness of the night, and the shrill chirping of crickets. His sleeping grandson's soft breathing was delightful to his ears. Suddenly, he felt human and alive, his heart touched in an unbelievable way.

Rediscovering your childhood spirit will connect you and make you live the present.

| 37 |

| THE FLEDGLING |

SELF-CONFIDENCE

"I developed my skills
after my many failures;
my existence, by my achievements.
It is all an art".

Vincent Cespedes

A peasant found an eagle's egg. He thought it belonged to one of his hens, so he placed it in the poultry-yard.

The young bird hatched among the hens. It learnt to walk like a hen, to cackle like a hen, and even to forage for food like a hen.

One day as it was busy foraging, its attention was attracted by a shadow high up in the sky: he saw a large and majestic bird soaring in the sky.

— What bird is that? Asked the little eagle that had been brought up among farm chickens.

— It's an eagle, he was informed. It's the largest and the swiftest of all birds!

The little eagle imagined how wonderful it must be to be able to soar high up in the sky. However, he thought he could never become an eagle, so he soon forgot about his dream and went about foraging for food as usual.

He lived his whole life believing he was a farmyard chicken, not knowing that he had the ability to soar in the sky like the eagle he had so admired.

Our innate abilities

are unlimited,

but we often prefer to limit

ourselves to our immediate thoughts..

| 38 |

| SUCH GREEN GRASS |

NO EFFORT, NO EXPECTATIONS

"Things get finished due to a lack of stability".

Pete Dexter

Two Ibex antelopes meet at the bottom of the valley. The first animal, full of pride and prancing around as if he was among females, tells the other:

— You can't beat me to the top.

— You think so? Says the second in a dreary tone.

— I'm the fastest and strongest Ibex in the whole area. I'll challenge you to a race to prove this: we need to get to the summit high above. The grass there is greener and delicious. Whoever arrives there first will have it all to himself.

— It's a bet.

The first Ibex shoots off at high speed. He climbs rapidly in an effort to be the first to arrive and retain his status among the rest of the Ibex.

His rival also sets off, but in a more relaxed manner. He maintains a trotting pace and keeps the other at close sight.

The proud Ibex finally arrives at the summit after a whole day of climbing like mad: he is completely exhausted after using up all his energy galloping at high speed. He falls to the ground, totally exhausted. An hour later, the second animal reaches the summit at a lively and measured pace. He is still spirited enough to tell the other:

— I didn't understand that the aim of the challenge was to be the first to arrive. Just look at yourself: yes, you arrived before me, but you're not even able to stand on your feet, let alone graze on the grass. As for me, let me enjoy myself.

In life, he who works with care

enjoys the fruits of his labor more

than he who charges on to exhaustion.

| 39 |

| A LIFE SAVED |

ACTING CONSCIOUSLY

"Altruism does not refer to merely performing acts of goodwill every now and then, it means always being compassionate and concerned about the well-being of others".

Jean-François Ricard

One day, a certain man was taking a walk along the street. Dark clouds in the sky covered the sun, and it soon started to rain heavily. Several snails, attracted by the humid weather, came up to take advantage of the unexpected windfall. Within a short time, the whole street was covered in shells.

The man strolled on despite the rain, and he soon saw a small boy beside the street: he was removing the snails one by one from the street and placing them with a lot of care beside the road. He worked on with a lot of enthusiasm.

— Young man, what are you doing? Asked the man. He was amazed at the boy who kept running around in all directions.

— I'm saving the snails from being crushed.

— That's crazy: just look, they're all over. You'll never be able to save them all. And the passersby are not even taking care where they walk… you're wasting your time…

Nevertheless, the boy still went on working: he came next to the man and picked up a snail that was near his feet, and cried out:

— For this one, I've not wasted my time!

The man's conscience was challenged by the child's openness and wisdom.

An unselfish act

is worth more than idle talk.

Altruism is an invaluable quality.

| 40 |

| THE DESIRE TO SEE LIFE AS IT IS |

ACCEPTANCE

"All flowers rush
to bequeath their lives,
their colors and their innocence to us.
Relishing their beauty brings perfection to life".

Christian Bobin

There was never a more pessimistic person that had ever lived. He was an intelligent and assertive man, full of mockery and irony. When he smoked his cigarettes, he would quietly blow out the smoke in long twirls, and thereafter buttonhole you with a chilling story about life. He did not see any good in anything: to him, all people were idiots, pleasures were vain, children, unbearable, the future, unreal, and fate, hollow... He denied everything that could be great, simple or beautiful.

One evening as he lay down to send a last heart-breaking SMS to a friend (*"Stop wishing me goodnight all the time. Spending the night in bed can never be good, that's where most people die"*), an opalescent ghost appeared before him, floating in the air:

— Aha!... Here I am at last! Cried out the ghost.

The man, teeth chattering, asked the ghost what he wanted...

— I've come to help you. You've complained for a very long time about human existence that we've decided to grant you nothingness from tonight.

— What? Cried out the man. But... no, not at all.... I don't want...!

— For a long time you have had a negative attitude towards everything, you have been pessimistic about everything... Death will surely be a welcome thing for you...!

Suddenly the man realized in all sincerity what he would lose and requested for his death to be postponed to a later time.

Life may probably not be perfect,

but it should be accepted

and lived as it is.

| 41 |

| WHAT IS GOOD, WHAT IS EVIL |

IMPARTIALITY

"After having lived one way or the other,
it would not be a bad idea to spend
around ten years or so seeing how others live,
laughing up your sleeve at their foolishness and saying:
"I'm not faring any better, but I understand them all".

Victor Cherublike (1880)

A tourist went to visit a country far away. He discovered that they had very strange and shocking behaviors, and opened up to his host about them:

— In my country, it's a very serious thing to make fun of and blaspheme against God.

— That's not the case in ours, replied his host.

— Criticizing the king is prohibited in my country.

— In ours it's not.

— Women are free in our country and they are allowed to put on make-up.

— That's not the case in ours.

— In our country, the right to own property is private and sacrosanct.

— Not in ours: anyone is free to own or not, to share or not.

— Education for children is a priority in our country: truancy is considered a bad thing.

— In ours, children are free to explore the world on their own and have personal experiences. It is considered a bad thing to force them into a system that is not convenient for them.

After spending a few more days of new discoveries, our tourist went back to his country, better informed about differences in viewpoints.

Good or evil,

are all relative

in terms of

place

or of time.

| 42 |

| THE GOD WHO COULD NOT SLEEP |

THE VIRTUES OF PATIENCE

"People react to anger like mirrors. That is the way their reflective neurons behave. These are cognitive structures where learning occurs by imitation. The same way a child mimics the facial reactions of its parents. Anger can contaminate an entire crowd".

Patrick Bauwen

An old legend tells of a god who felt that he was not being recognized for his true worth, nor was he seated at his proper position in the court of the palace of the gods.

Day and night he fussed about his situation, pondering endlessly in between fits of anger and underhand dealings.

He gained the reputation of being the least consulted of all the gods. Instead of calming down, he became more demanding, banging his fist on the table during meetings, claiming to being treated with injustice and a lack of due recognition.

— See how you all treat me badly! I'm superior to many of you here! I need not justify myself to any of you!

He could no longer sleep as a result of his anger. He would wake up every night and pace up and down for hours on end. All alone in his temple-house up in the skies, the others had simply kept him in isolation. He remained in this state, his heart full of rage, for centuries on end. Nobody came to see him anymore. Human beings even forgot his name.

Until the day he acknowledged his error and said to himself: “I’ve lost everything; I no longer have a position among the gods. Humans don’t even know me anymore”.

Once his bitterness was gone, he was able to fall asleep for the first time. His nights became so peaceful henceforth he became known as “the Morpheus god”.

Unjustified anger cannot bring inner peace or lead to personal advancement. It is a destructive force to anyone who harbors it. Releasing your anger brings inner peace.

| 43 |

| THE ROAD |

THE VIRTUES OF PATIENCE

"People gave consideration
only to the departure and arrival points
and ignored the road
that linked the two".

Yann Apperry

Convinced of his facts, a cheetah teased a gazelle:

— I'm the fastest of all animals.

— If you say so, replied the gazelle.

— I'll give you a challenge if you don't believe me: we'll race to the top of the mountain over there. I eat you if you lose.

— I don't by any means have any other choice but to accept.

The cheetah leapt ahead: he ran off at full speed. The gazelle, on his part, left trotting. He came across a zebra whose hoof was wedged in a hole and helped him get it out.

He met a lion along the way to the top of the mountain and talked to him briefly. He also met with a snake and other animals as well. Finally, he helped a buffalo find her calf who had strayed.

The cheetah was obviously the first to arrive at their destination:

— I've been waiting for the past three days. I haven't had anything to eat, and since I've proved that I'm faster, I'm going to eat you, he added, even though he was exhausted.

However, all the animals that the gazelle had helped along the way appeared at that moment:

— You may be the fastest animal, but you'll not touch a single fur of our dear friend, they all said in unison.

Rushing is not winning. The route you take in your life and the people you meet are more important than hurrying with the desire to win. We are all going to the same destination, it is thus preferable to make the journey more interesting.

| 44 |

| IN A RIVER |

A NEW MINDSET

"When your mind becomes unbalanced,
away from your comfort zone,
your usual habits,
perhaps that is the time to take a step back for
a moment of reflection.
You could use the opportunity to think over
your life, for introspection,
to cogitate over your state of mind.
When reading a book,
try to meditate over what it is about
and identify the feelings
and new ideas it is arousing in you.
We rarely have the time for all that.
We should thus relish
these moments of leisure".

Frédéric Lenoir

Two fish were swimming leisurely and enjoying the calm, clear waters of a river. They swam back and forth through the slow currents, gliding among the algae, or hiding in holes next to the river bank in between the roots.

— I love this place, said the first fish. I know it very well.

— Of course not, retorted the second.

— That's not true! I was born here, and this river is my home!

— You only know a part of it. On the other side of the mirror is an entirely different world you know nothing of (he was referring to the land).

— That's not important! I know MY territory very well: I know where to get the tastiest algae, where the fry swim, or where the flies get trapped…

— That may be so, I agree that this place is always peaceful. But the water we swim in isn't always the same. Sometimes it is fresh, other times it is disturbed, at times calm, another time scarce… There's always something new you learn about this river, the same way you have to find out every day where the fisherman is trying to trap us.

The first fish could not find anything to say, instead he set to think over these words of wisdom.

Leaving your comfort zone enables you to discover new experiences, and you will be able to avoid going round in circles.

| 45 |

| MAKING CHOICES IN LIFE AT EVERY OPPORTUNITY |

SELF-CONFIDENCE

"Avoid placing unnecessary
mental beacons all over.
You will never go wrong by following your instincts. Birds
migrate every year
without knowing why.
Well, it will be for our good if we did the same,
always on the move,
without asking too many questions".

Lorenzo Marone

It was total devastation in the forest: it had never rained so heavily in animal memory! The birds hid in tree boughs, the rabbits in burrows and the wild boars in the undergrowth. From their hiding places, the animals could see the little mouse walking in the rain…

— Mouse, where are you going in this horrible weather?

— I'm going to the top of the hill where I'll be better off.

— You must be mad! The rain will soak you!

The mouse walked on without paying attention to the animals.

At the edge of the forest, he came across some cows, goats and sheep huddled together to avoid the icy rain. They asked him:

— Mouse, where are you going in this horrible weather?

— I'm going to the top of the hill where I'll be better off.

— You must be mad! You'll freeze in the rain!.

The mouse walked on and soon arrived at the top of the hill. From the high land he could see the devastation of the lowland, farms soaked in water, with the raindrops on the forest leaves giving out a shiny hue. But he felt safe where he was. It rained heavily the entire night.

The following morning, he could see nothing but water all around him...: the flood had swept away the animals, and the trees, uprooted by the muddy waters, had all fallen. Thanks to his decision to listen only to his inner voice, he was the only one whose life had been spared.

Every moment of your life is an opportunity:

the choices that we make

will determine the path it takes.

| 46 |

| I WANT |

NO EFFORT, NO EXPECTATIONS

"Anticipating the future in the mind
gives us three unique abilities:
to foresee, to desire, and to prepare".

Jean-Louis Servan-Schreiber

A legend in a certain village had it that whoever caught a red fish in the neighboring river would become immensely rich. All children were told this tale. Everybody knew this was a story that children were told at their bedtimes.

However, one of them made a firm decision to catch this fish.

— I want to catch the red fish. I want to be rich.

Several years passed by. The amused laughter of the villagers turned to open mockery at the boy who grew up to become an adolescent, an adult, and finally an old man. Every day, he went to the river with a fishing line, and walked along the bank in search of the legendary red fish that was nothing but a village tale.

Any time anyone tried to reason with him, he would reply:

— I want this fish and I'll get it! I'll not give up! You'll all see!

As time passed by with no luck on his side, he would now only reply:

— I want. I want. I want.

He spent his whole life this way till his last day. He never stopped believing what his mind told him, believing in the story. His selfish desire had deceived him: he had fixed his mind so much on the legend that he ended up spending his entire life in vain.

Desiring something at all cost is an illusion of our minds: this reduces the capacity of our minds to reason, making us miss opportunities that come up in our lives.

| 47 |

| THE BURDEN |

ACTING CONSCIOUSLY

"Rain re-focuses our attention to our thoughts.
We do not look at other passersby when it rains;
we walk with our heads bowed,
eyes fixed on restless puddles of water".

Karen Maitland

One day, two gentlemen arrived at a certain town. It was buzzing with activity. In front of a hotel at the central square, a lady was waiting for assistance to climb down from a sedan-chair.

The rain had left behind open pools of dirty water mixed with mud. The lady could not cross them without soiling her long and expensive dress that gave an indication of her wealthy background. She sat silently, irritated and very annoyed; she would not stop scolding her servants.

However, they were in confusion: They were carrying her boxes in their hands. They could not put them down on the dirty ground, or risk them being stolen.

The younger of the two gentlemen looked at the lady, and walked on without saying a word. The older one, on his part, walked towards the lady, carried her in his arms, crossed the pools of water and let her down on the other side of the street.

The lady dismissed him without a word, turned around and walked away in open pride. Her servants followed her to avoid fanning her anger any further.

Our two gentlemen continued on their way. The younger one could not help thinking about the incident over and over in his mind. After a few hours, he could no longer contain himself and shouted out:

— That lady was really contemptuous and offensive! You helped her to cross over the pools of water, yet she did not even utter a word of thanks. What a shame! And you're not even her valet.

— I assisted the lady several hours ago, replied his companion. Why are you still bothered and continuing to carry her in your mind?

It serves no purpose worrying about the past: it just poisons the present.

| 48 |

| ARCHIBALD AND THE CYCLE OF LIFE |

ACCEPTANCE

"Allowing my body become dust
and humus without a fuss, fattening worms,
and providing nourishment for plants, letting life
go its full cycle.
That is the only form of eternity
that I can hope for".

André Brink

A long time ago in a small village, there lived an old man named Archibald. He refused to die and had postponed his death so many times, he was thus not worried when it came for him once more one night.

— Is it you again, you flathead? Asked the old man.

— Archibald, please be reasonable and just agree to die.

— No! I'm against death and will not agree to die. There's no discussion about that.

— Nevertheless, you do it every day…

— That's not true! I'm against it and will never kill! Shouted the old man, offended.

— Every single day, your body kills thousands of bacteria to survive. You destroy germs, red and white blood cells… just so you can continue living… Your life depends on death.

— Of course, not! Germs attack me, I have to defend myself!

— True… but what about the food you eat? Every meal you take means that plants and animals had to be sacrificed, and these are living things…

— But… all I'm doing is to transform them…

— You'll also be transformed…

— Just a minute! The old man cried out in panic. What about you? How is it that you never die? That's not fair.

— Actually, that's true. I don't die. And do you know why?

— No.

— Because I don't exist. You are alive, so, for you, death isn't real. You can't feel or see it. But when you die, I shall no longer exist for you either.

The old man Archibald mulled over this. It is said that the following morning he was found gone with a peaceful smile on his face.

Life is a cycle and it serves no purpose trying to go against this. You need to accept and let it to make its full circle.

| 49 |

| TRAPPED BY THE MIND |

IMPARTIALITY

"Failure is first a feeling,
long before becoming a reality.
It is the result of a combination between vulnerability and a lack of self-confidence,
and is thereafter made worse,
often deliberately, by fear".

Michelle Obama

It was Justine's big day. She was supposed to have an audition for her certification as an acoustic guitar player following her studies at the conservatoire. She had been born surrounded by guitars. Her father was an accomplished guitarist.

She, too, was talented, but pressure piled up on her as her D-day approached. A silent voice kept whispering in her mind: "What if I don't make it?"; "I've a feeling that I'm going to fail"; "I fear that I'm going to disappoint my father"; "I'm not up to the mark".

All the same, the test was a piece she knew very well. But she found the looks on the faces of the jury, her parents' presence and her worries over failing more and more disconcerting.

Indeed, she was very uncomfortable when she climbed up on stage. Her whole mind was gripped by the fear of failing.

She had programmed herself for failure. After three attempts, her fingers trembling, she could not play beyond a few chords. The jury politely thanked her and requested her to leave and let the next candidate to come in.

Justine walked out, totally disappointed: “I knew I wouldn’t make the mark”. She burst into tears.

We pay too much attention to this inner voice that keeps judging and discouraging us. Which failures in your life are a result of this?

| 50 |

| THE POWER OF SILENCE |

THE VIRTUES OF PATIENCE

"I owe my success in overcoming silence to books.
They are like passports.
They break down walls, ramparts, boundaries and all manner of barriers invented by mankind for their self-isolation and heartbreak".

Irene Frain

Several important political changes were expected in a small kingdom hidden away in the Himalayan mountains. King Atsong was expected to appoint his head of government. Two candidates presented themselves for the post, but each had totally different policies and ideas for governing the kingdom. Calang was of the opinion that the caste and hierarchy system currently in force should be continued. Hyen, on the other hand, felt that this social system was paralyzing the country's development and should be relaxed.

Calang was called in first, given that he had for long been close to the royal family. The king informed him as soon as he entered the office:

— I need to appoint one of you as the Prime Minister, said the king, in the hope that Hyen could be persuaded to support his rival.

This however did not take place. The latter did not utter a word. The room became quiet for ten seconds, then twenty seconds, and finally forty.

— May I please ask if I can confirm to Mr. Calang that you agree to become a member of his cabinet?

The office was silent for more than a minute. Calang was visibly uncomfortable. The silence was so heavy he finally cracked and said out loud:

— No! No! It's not fair to ask that of Mr. Hyen. He should be the one appointed to this post.

Patience and silence

are more important

than haste and agitation.

| 51 |

| WOMAN IN A RUSH |

THE VIRTUES OF PATIENCE

"Intelligence is the ability to establish links between the absolutes that our experiences present to us".

Michel Tournier

She gripped her fingers on the steering wheel so hard that her fists turned white. The traffic jam was unbearable, and it racked her nerves. Negative thoughts raced through her mind about the tasks she had ahead of her: she would have to push the children take their bath in a hurry, she would have to prepare dinner in a rush, she was not going to have the time to call her mother as she had planned to, she would not have a little time to relax before putting the children to bed…

She tried to take another route, but it was equally as bad as the main one. She had the desire to press hard on the car horn. She accelerated quickly as soon as some space opened up, and stopped twenty meters ahead. She felt that she had done all she could to move fast.

She was literally a nervous wreck when she arrived at the child-care center. All was well, the children had been playing without kicking up a fuss. She huddled them into the car and left in a rush. She washed them quickly and made them eat their dinner under a tense atmosphere.

It was not until after the children had gone to sleep that she finally realized how her evening and her mood had been ruined by her impatience to get back home quickly. If she had only accepted the reality that she would be arriving home late, if she had imagined the pleasure of seeing her children rather than worry about the impossibility of arriving at a time she felt was "normal", her whole evening would have ended up totally different.

Our impatience

is usually the source

of our discomfort.

| 52 |

| THE WONDER IN YOU |

A NEW MINDSET

"Curiosity as you understand it,
is it not essentially an art?
The art of selecting? The art of navigating?
The art of living? The art of traveling at low cost? A remedy to indifference?
A desire to see for yourself,
to read with no restrictions, to keep asking
questions all the time about existence,
and not losing so soon
the liveliness of childhood?
A way of being alive, and feeling alive
to the end of your days on earth?"

Jean-Pierre Martin

Can you imagine one day, one morning, being replaced by the person you were as a child? Can you imagine the child you used to be, coming to your house, your apartment and using your furniture? Can you imagine this child driving your car all alone, or taking the subway to go to your place of work? Try to imagine his or her surprise and admiration when they start carrying out your daily responsibilities and discovering what you have always taken to be usual and normal.

Perhaps you have not been happy with your life and achievements, especially the invariability and relentlessness that is part and parcel of today's life.

However, it would be important to rediscover the child in you, the person you once were: a small child, yes, but fresh and new in spirit, and ready to be amazed at everything.

Take time to allow
the child in you to tell you,
from their viewpoint, all that you are doing,
everything that is good,
positive and pleasant about your life.

| 53 |

| THE POTTER |

SELF-CONFIDENCE

"There is something extraordinarily fake, paradoxical and almost unreal about the work of a nurse, when seen from a medical psychology viewpoint.
The more the nurse follows the rules, the less they need to think, gradually losing the power of intuition, repressing their feelings and taking patients as objects.
The better they get as 'nurses', the less they become as 'caregivers'".

Roger Gentis

One fine day, an honorable potter found a piece of Chinese ceramic… Even though he had worked with clay for many years, he was very impressed by the delicateness, the brilliance and the purity of the masterpiece that he was holding in his hands! He was so mesmerized by it that he resolved to find out for himself the secret of his fellow artisan from the other end of the world.

Our potter thus set out, every single day without fail, to test and try all kinds of materials, tools, colors and oven temperatures. Soon, his relentlessness at the work spread all over that people started to take him for a madman.

One day he went to his shed to look for firewood to make his fire hotter, but found it empty. He had used up all his firewood! The artisan decided to go into his house and took his table, saying: “Our food will taste even better if we eat from the floor”.

But the fire was still not getting hot enough, so he went for his chairs. He said: “Food will taste even much better when eaten squatting”.

The fire got hotter, but not as much as our good man wanted. He got hold of his axe, and soon his wardrobe was reduced to pieces of wood. He said: “Who needs a wardrobe when you have no chairs?”.

He finally discovered the secret he had been searching for: he discovered that the hotter the fire, the finer the piece of ceramic.

Is this not such a beautiful lesson?

Especially given that this is a true story,

and that the artisan who followed his intuition

was called Bernard Palissy.

Never ignore your intuition:

it can be your guide.

| 54 |

| NEGATIVE FEELINGS |

ACTING CONSCIOUSLY

"In order to grow, wheat requires sunshine,
and beetroot needs rain.
this makes sense, and gives the farmer
the reason to complain about
the weather regardless of the season".

Jean-Louis Fournier

The gentleman was mad at everything. He was even mad at being mad.

It is true that his day had been terrible indeed. To start with, he had spent hours on end stuck in traffic, and he only managed to arrive at work on time after driving like mad once it opened up. Thereafter, he got terribly upset by his colleagues for their utter inefficiency and inability to understand his ideas, or even do anything useful. The lunch at the restaurant was cold and his favorite dessert was not done as liked it. His evening was ruined by a long meeting that only wasted his time. He tried to busy himself by taking endless cups of coffee and smoking one cigarette after the other.

He was a total wreck by the time he got back home in the evening.

It had indeed been a bad day.

As if that was not bad enough, it began to rain. He furiously turned on the windscreen wipers. It seemed that the end of his misery was not in sight yet!

He noticed an electric wheelchair in front of him as he turned on to the road leading to his neighborhood.

He recognized the silhouette of his young neighbor who was temporarily confined to a wheelchair following an operation after a spinal injury. She'll probably need to use it for the rest of her life, he thought to himself. He overtook her, and by instinct looked back through the rearview mirror.

It was her, a young lady that he hardly knew anything about.

There was a flash of lightning, and the gentleman saw the young woman smiling. Her eyes were turned up towards the sky, and raindrops fell on her face. She relished being outdoors, able to move about, to be alive and savoring the ambience.

Suddenly the gentleman began to ask himself if he had really done anything worthwhile the whole day.

We are all at liberty to react to our situations: do we choose to live our lives with joy or in boredom filled with endless complaints?

| 55 |

| THE MAYFLY |

ACCEPTANCE

"Loving abundantly and living abundantly.
Loving forever and living forever.
Eternal life is attached to Love".

Paulo Coelho

A mayfly was flying around in the bright daylight. It had been alive for the last ten hours, and it could feel its end approaching. It perched on a leaf and started lamenting:

— What a sad life I'm living! I've spent half of my life learning about myself, only to realize that I know almost nothing… then I have to prepare to die. If only I could live as long as a bird…

At that moment it noticed a tit perched on a branch. It was an avid eater of gnats, and it was lamenting:

— I've been living on this earth for almost three years now… my children are all grown up and soon I'll be dead and gone for good! Oh, what a sad life! There's still so much I need to learn about the world and life… there's still a lot I need to enjoy… If only I could live for as long as the tortoise…!

At that moment a tortoise passed by. It is one of the longest living animals on earth, but it was also groaning:

— One hundred and twenty years! What's that compared to the life of the stars… How sad it is that I can never live for as long as they do…

Just like mayflies, stars also end up dying. The best thing to do is to accept things as they are if we have no control over them. We too, like suns, flowers and galaxies, will all die one day. So why should we waste our time and lives worrying about death?

| 56 |

| THE TRUTH IN WRONG |

IMPARTIALITY

"Is not allowing
what refuses to be silenced in me
to speak out, the most natural way
to be human and simple?
I shall not be forced to lie
in order to appear to be sincere according to man".

Marcel Arland

In an inn in the Netherlands. It is the year 1578. Two friends are having a passionate discussion about the most recent scientific discoveries over a cup of coffee with milk:

— The earth is round and is at the center of the universe.

— That's utter nonsense! It's obvious that the earth is flat and the sun is at the center of the universe.

You're completely mistaken. Remember Magellan? Didn't he travel around the world by ship to prove that indeed the earth is round?

— That doesn't prove anything. What about Copernicus? Didn't he say that the earth turns around the sun? You can't disparage the findings of such a scientist that you, too, respect a lot..

The discussion became so animated that it finally degenerated into a fistfight, to the amusement of the other clients. The two friends had to be separated in the end.

— You're such an idiot, said one to the other.

— You're the idiot in this case, replied the other.

A very close friendship completely destroyed. Who was right? Who was wrong?

None of them, and both of them at the same time. But what was more important?

| 57 |

| THE SACRED WAVE |

THE VIRTUES OF PATIENCE

*"Assuming a tenacious appearance
and a liberated identity
can only be achieved by acknowledging that we are but mere mediators, and knowing that we are not any more real or have a better fate than a wave in the ocean".*

Nicolas Grimaldi

A story is told in the Pacific islands of a tribal prince who was fascinated by waves. His father informed him:

— You shall become the chief if you manage to tame Uluhia, the sacred wave.

This referred to an enormous wave that crashed the coastline every five to seven years. It was so terrifying that everybody was awed by it.

From that moment the prince always walked along the coastline in the hope of encountering this natural phenomenon from the ocean. He went to the beach every single day of the week in the desire to discover the secret of the wave. At first, he went out in a canoe, but it soon broke up. He realized that a long plank of wood allowed him more mobility and freedom of movement. Nonetheless, he could not discover anything. He got swept away by a surge in the ocean when he approached it. The day of Uluhia finally arrived. The prince had grown to a young man. The tide had moved far enough, a sign of the coming of the giant wave.

He watched the horizon keenly the evening before, with an anxious look on his face. He was aware that, as the son of the chief, the following day would be his encounter with fate under the watchful eye of his father. But he was equally aware that he had not yet achieved his victory. He had used up a lot of his strength in his quest, but each time the ocean had triumphed over him. His attention was attracted by an albatross that had landed a little far off in the ocean. A wave was approaching, and the son of the chief feared that the bird would be swallowed by it. To his big surprise, this did not happen; the albatross did not dive to escape the wave, but instead let itself be carried along, keeping in rhythm with its undulating movement. The son of the chief cried out:

— I've found out how to overcome Uluhia! I don't need to attack or fight it, but move with it and let it carry me along as a friend.

Life is like this wave: sometimes terrifying and worrying; you will not find peace if you confront these times head-on and face to face. You need to accept and move along with them in order to gain a measure of control: you need to surf along with life, not against it.

| 58 |

| THE PRESENT TIME |

A NEW MINDSET

"Everything will fade away, time, clouds in the sky, human life, all move from birth towards their death. Do not become emotionally dependent on the passage of time, it is not the best way to view the world. Make every second of your life count, without getting worried of the past days and mornings that will never come back. The present time is the only thing without an end".

An American-Indian Proverb

Two managers are having a discussion as they stand beside a coffee dispenser:

— I've a meeting at 11, then I need to go and buy myself a sandwich. I'll have about thirty minutes to eat it, and thereafter I have to take my car to the garage. I come back for another meeting. After that I have twenty minutes to go and buy some bread and to pick up my children at 5pm. Finally, I'll be back home to prepare for…

Suddenly he stops speaking in mid-sentence…

— What a terrible day!... I'm stressed…

His colleague remains silent.

— How do you manage to stay so calm all the time? We both attend meetings and have similar lifestyles.

— Oh, well, I don't really do anything special.

— That can’t be. But tell me,… is it that your wife does everything for you? Do you take vitamin pills? Tell me what you do to remain always composed like that.

— None of those. I just do things when they should be done. When it’s time for work, I work; the time for walking, I walk; the time for driving, I drive; the time for cooking, I cook…

His colleague looks at him in amazement. Some people say that time is a silent destroyer that kills you in the end. They thus rush in desperation to do as much as possible every second of their lives. On the other hand, you could choose to consider every second as significant, even though time flies. Each second should be appreciated for what it brings.

Each second of your life

is a gift,

that is why

it is called “the present”.

| 59 |

| BECOMING YOURSELF |

SELF-CONFIDENCE

"You do not lose anything by being what you already are.
We are aware of what is important in life,
and what you can gain in the world.
You should only concentrate on being yourself.
Discovering yourself is the key".

Frédérique Deghelt

Once upon a time a raven and his wife were impatiently waiting for their eggs to hatch. Finally, the eggshells started moving about and breaking one after the other. eventually five chicks were hatched. One of them was smaller than the rest and had a tiny beak. No matter, said his father. We shall feed him well and he will grow fast.

Indeed, the parents did not spare any efforts in feeding their chicks.

They began to teach them all that was required to become a raven, especially how to caw whenever dark clouds hang low over the countryside.

The chicks grew and the quicker ones soon started developing black feathers. To the surprise of the parents, they noticed that the last, the smallest one, started developing red feathers instead of black! Not only that, he did not grow as quickly as the others, his feathers never turned black, and worst of all, he could not learn to caw!

The little red one, as they all called him, soon gave up trying to grow as big as his brothers; he was convinced he would never be able to do it.

He also gave up trying to learn to caw as the others; he knew this was impossible.

But he decided to do something with his high-pitched voice. He would sing from morning till evening.

Once he stopped trying to be a raven, he turned out to be a wonder to behold.

Soon the truth became more evident. He resembled a robin more than a raven, and everyone accepted him as he was.

Eventually he became the most beautiful bird in the entire woodland with the sweetest singing voice.

Do not allow anyone to tell you what to be: just be yourself.

That is your greatest inner strength.

| 60 |

| THE MAN AND THE BIRD |

ACTING CONSCIOUSLY

"Every single person,
no matter how much they
are in control of their feelings,
will soon reveal them in one way or the other".

Dean Koontz

An Arab tale tells of a man who once caught a very frail bird. It was so small it could fit in the palm of his hand. The bird tried to plead with the man for its freedom:

— What can you get from me? It said. I'm so tiny and frail, I'm just skin and bones! Please let me go! I'll tell you three truths in exchange.

— Agreed, said the man. But how will I know if these truths are useful to me?

— It's very simple. I'll tell you the first truth while you're still holding me in your hand. I shall tell you the second one while I'm on the branch of that tree; that way, you'll still be able to catch me if the truth isn't convenient to you. Finally, I shall tell you the third, the most important one, while I'm soaring high up in the sky.

— Fine, replied the man. Tell me the first one.

— You should not regret it if you lose anything, even though it be your own life.

That's such a profound truth, said the man: it's about not being attached to worldly things, the secret to true freedom. He opened the palm of his hand. The bird flew to the branch, and said the second truth:

— Never believe anyone telling you any kind of nonsense, unless they can prove it beforehand.

— Very good! Said the man. You are wiser than your bird-brain seems to indicate: human beings are in reality naturally attracted by lies and illusions due to greed! So, what is the third truth?

— In my stomach I've two large diamonds, each as big as your fist, said the bird as it flew high up in the sky. You'd have become very rich if you'd decided to kill me.

The man cursed at the bird in rage. He blamed himself for having been so stupid and wept about his fate.

— Idiot! Exclaimed the bird. I told you never to regret anything, and you're already regretting having released me!

I told you not to believe any absurdity, and you believed me, tiny as I am and fitting in one palm of your hand, that I had swallowed two diamonds, each as large as your fist!

Due to your greed and stupidity, you'll never be able to fly high in the sky like I do.

Our own feelings can easily have a negative impact on our best principles and beliefs. Could this be the time to stop them from having any influence on our lives?

| 61 |

| THE MAN WITH DIFFERENT COLORED EYES |

IMPARTIALITY

"No matter how ordinary it may be, my beauty does not need your empty praises: beauty lies in the eyes of the beholder, not in humiliating praise of the tongue whose only interest is to boast".

William Shakespeare

People always looked at Peter "crosswise" ever since his birth, in a manner of speaking. He was born with different colored eyes, that is, one blue eye, while the other was very dark brown, almost black.

This affected him a lot since he was a child and it made him feel different. The other children also stayed away from him. In his youth, he was rejected several times by the girls he approached, who described him as "rather strange", or "he looks like a sort of a monster".

Peter was not yet married by the time he reached 40 years old. He believed that the different colors of his eyes made him look ugly. He took it for granted and considered that, despite his age and experience, his strange eyes were a prior disqualification for any relationship.

To celebrate his 40th birthday, he decided to take a holiday in a paradise island in the Pacific Ocean. Peter was taken aback by what was happening as soon as he alighted from the plane: all the women were smiling at him, and from all evidence, they were all desiring to hold his hand.

Many women were making advances at him in the streets. He could not understand what was going on. It was the first time he was understanding his power of seduction.

Finally, a resident explained it to him:

— Local legend has it that any person with eyes of different colors is a protégé of our traditional god. In our culture, you are thus associated with prosperity, beauty and goodwill. Don't be surprised therefore by the reaction of our women!

Having thus discovered that he was such a "seductive man", he decided to settle on the island, eventually starting a family with a woman he fell in love with and married.

By viewing our physical selves through our personal judgements and through others' eyes, we ignore our inner and outer beauty, as well as our seductive potential.

| 62 |

| A MATTER OF PERCEPTION |

THE VIRTUES OF PATIENCE

"Perception is not a science of the world,
it is not even an act,
or a deliberate point of view taken,
it is the foundation on which all acts differ, one from the other, and which they all take for granted".

Maurice Merleau-Ponty

Two friends on their way from the cinema.

— What a film! It's so touching, this story of a naïve footballer who gets exploited by the system and those around him.

— I loved it. I found it funny and refreshing.

— Funny? Continued his friend. I didn't find it funny at all. It was touching, and even sad… how can you find the fate of this innocent man to be funny?

— Well, I don't know: I found him to be rather a silly clown; he reminded me of Charlie Chaplin. It was quite amusing the way he moved around clumsily. To me, there was nothing sad or touching about him at all.

— The end was very bad for him: he is sacked from the team and he becomes a totally unknown fruit seller, whereas he could have become a famous football star.

— Exactly, but he seems to be happier in the end: he did not achieve the glory he had hoped for, but he is smiling in the last scene…

One film, same story, but with two different points of view. The same thing occurs in real life: your life and the perceptions you have of it are personal and subjective. Nothing is absolute.

How do you react to each experience in your life?

What point of view will you take?

| 63 |

| PRAISE FOR CHANGE |

A NEW MINDSET

"Living is losing...
We can live a happier life if we can adapt
and accept that nothing
is permanent and
that change is inevitable".

Louise Penny

A caterpillar was crawling painfully on a branch. It felt tired and was aware that its time was almost up.

— Alas! Soon I'll be dead and stuffed like a dry piece of hide.

Its mind reeled back to its past: its encounters, the feasting on tender green leaves, the enjoyable rainy days.

— I wish everything could remain as they were before, that nothing would change. If only time could stand still.

A butterfly came towards the caterpillar, attracted by its lamenting.

— Why are you lamenting so much?

— Well, I'm so sad that I'm soon leaving this world.

— But why are you cursing changes and sticking onto fixation? Everything is always on the move and changing. You should have a flexible mind that is willing to embrace change rather than remain fixed on illusions.

— But I don't want to end up immobile on this branch. I would have been happier crawling all my life and not feeling sorry for myself.

— Are you aware that soon you will transform into a butterfly with beautiful wings for flying around?

Embracing change, rather than going against it and sticking to the past, is the best way of allowing the best opportunities to come into your life.

| 64 |

| THE PRINCE'S GARDEN |

SELF-CONFIDENCE

"Sight is perhaps always influenced, and it relies on one's ability to compare one thing from another".

Vidiadhar Surajprasad Naipaul

A certain prince planted around his castle all kinds of trees, plants and flowers. It was a very large and beautiful garden. He took a walk every day, enjoying the fresh air around his home. One day he left on a journey, and when he returned, the first thing that he did was to take a walk around his garden. Sadly, he found that the trees and plants were drying up. He was greatly affected by this, and reflected on the past magnificence of his garden. He asked a weeping willow what could have led to this bad state. The tree informed him:

— I took one look at the pear tree and realized I'll never be able to produce such beautiful fruits. I became discouraged and started to dry up.

The prince went on in search of the pear tree. It, too, was dying. He asked it what was wrong and it answered:

— After seeing the rose plant and smelling its perfume, I knew I'll never be as refined and delicate. As a result, I started drying up, replied the fruit tree. The rose plant on its part was also wasting away. The prince went to inquire from it, and it said:

— I'd really love to live for as long as that maple tree. I wish my leaves did not have to dry up in autumn, and my petals to last a bit longer. But this can't be, so I let myself dry up.

The prince was getting annoyed, but he decided nonetheless to continue his walk. Suddenly, his sight was attracted by a beautiful little flower in full bloom. In surprise, he went to it to ask how it had remained so fresh.

— I, too, almost dried up. At first, I was getting discouraged since I knew I could never be as magnificent as a willow tree; nor be as delicate and sweet smelling as the rose plant. I began drying up, but I said to myself: if the prince, who is rich, powerful and wise, and who had planted this garden, had wanted anything else apart from me here, he would have planted it instead. If he had planted me, that means that he wanted me here as I am. I decided from then on to stop comparing myself to others, and bring out the best in me, for myself.

Our minds are often more inclined towards discouragement and comparison. It also ends up drying out. Love, confidence in, as well as high regard of yourself are the fertile grounds for nourishing your inner lives.

| 65 |

| THE MONKEY |

IMPARTIALITY

"The best form of wisdom is not to be wise".

Angelus Silesius

A certain man, after a failed relationship, decided to travel to India for a change of atmosphere, and also to be as far away as possible from the woman who had broken his heart so much.

He hoped this would enable him to relax and find some sort of inner peace. However, even while that far away, he could not help thinking of her all the time. Wherever he went, every single moment, at every turn of the street or whichever restaurant he went to, his mind was obsessed by the image of the woman who had so much captured his feelings. This left him feeling sad and morose at the same time. She had totally captured his heart and his mind as well.

He was overwhelmed by his feelings. He wished they were together in this foreign country.

One day as he was taking a stroll in the forest, along a path leading up a hill overhanging the town, he was lost in thought when he noticed a wise man meditating in the open air, near the path.

— Ah... If only I could be at peace like him...

The wise man opened his eyes and looked at the traveler. He considered this an invitation from the wise man and started talking to him.

— I really admire your peace of mind. What do you do to feel like this?

The wise man pointed towards a monkey passing by, wandering about and jumping from one branch to the other.

— The mind is like that monkey, always in motion, always active. That's how it is. When mine becomes agitated, I just let it wander around as it wishes. That's all.

Simply by observing our minds in a neutral and impartial way, we would be able to understand it better and, in so doing, avoid being confined by it.

| 66 |

| ALL ABOUT OVER-EXERTION |

THE VIRTUES OF PATIENCE

"Organization is not about putting things in order. It is all about giving life".

Jean-René Fourtou

A man is seated in the garden. His name is Martin. He is busy thinking over his life. He is almost at a dead-end. A manager in a large company, he has a huge backlog of work as the files keep piling up on his desk. He does not wish to disappoint his boss, but the work is wearing him down. He is unable to keep up the rhythm. Furthermore, he has to take care of his three children when he returns home in the evening. Yet he has to keep his job. He has no time for sports, or be with his friends... Yes, he is about to reach a dead-end. His life has become an accumulation of tasks to be performed, in silence, like a zombie. He is no longer happy. It is too much.... He can feel the burnout coming.

Martin was so carried away in his thoughts that he paid no attention to the birds singing or the winds blowing over the leaves. Suddenly his attention was attracted towards an old man sitting on a bench, smiling and preparing tea. His serenity as he prepared the tea made Martin move towards him.

— Hello, sir! You look so at ease sitting there, said he to the old man.

— The birds and the weather are equally calm, replied the old man as he continued preparing the tea.

— That's true… But personally, I'm not at peace… Have you ever felt that way? There's so much to be done at work… And I have three children…

Martin rolled out a long list of things that made his life unbearable.

— Here, said the old man as he offered Martin a cup of tea.

Our man hardly noticed offer and went on with his endless grumbling, until the cup spilled over as the old man poured the tea.

— Hold on! Stop! Cried out Martin.

— You, just like this cup, are overflowing with your own burdens and negative thoughts, said the old man. How can I be of any help to you unless you first empty your cup?

The way to acquiring self-control starts with learning to sort out your life and putting it in order.

| 67 |

| COMPLAINING |

A NEW MINDSET

"We pass judgement to everything
that happens in our lives,
we rejoice, and we complain.
However, it is only at the end that we shall know
if we should have rejoiced or complained.
Life is not rigid, it keeps changing."

Virginie Grimaldi

The devil came to the world with the desire to deceive mankind. He derived a lot of pleasure out of tormenting people. One day he met a poor shepherd and approached him, pretending to be a wise man.

— How are you, dear friend? He asked.

— Well, my kind old man, I'm not fine... I'm always faccd with onc difficulty or the other, always looking forward to the evening so I can get away from this tiresome work of pasturing sheep till the following morning. I look forward all the time to Midsummer Day and Christmas... at least then I can have a little fun. The devil smiled to himself. How gullible man can be! He removed a ball of wool from his pocket and said:

— Worry no more my dear shepherd! I have the solution to your problems, and as a friend, I'll give it to you. Here's a ball of wool. The day will come to an end in an instant if you unroll it a little. If you unroll it more, a month or an entire year will pass by under your eyes. You will no longer have to be waiting in vain!

— You'll give it to me? Really?

— Exactly! And with no strings attached. It's my pleasure if I can be of service.

And with that he left the ball of wool with the shepherd. The following morning, wishing to avoid the boredom of herding his sheep an entire day, the shepherd unrolled the ball a bit, and in an instant, it was evening. He was amazed at the realization that he could go back to bed immediately after having just woken up! The shepherd made it a habit to unroll the ball at the slightest excuse: whenever it rained, when the sun was too hot, when the holidays were taking too long to come, whenever he was troubled, whenever he was faced with challenges, or even whenever he felt lovesick. One day as he was about to pull on the string due to pain in his legs, he noticed that his fingers seemed aged, twisted and numb. The ball in his hand had also been reduced to just a small string.

His entire body started trembling, and he could swear that he heard a burst of laughter in the background.

Always complaining about your fate is the surest way to missing out on the best in your life.

| 68 |

| PREMATURE JUDGEMENT |

IMPARTIALITY

"Waves are nothing
in comparison to the whole ocean".

Claude Lelouch

A certain man and his son were standing by looking at the sea.

They had lived in the region their entire lives, and like everyone else in the village, they survived on crabs, shell-fish, algae and fish. They lived under a tough, cold and foggy environment. The sea at times was also rough and unfriendly. However, just like the shell-fish clinging onto rocks, the villagers continued living there.

— Tell me, daddy, asked the young boy.

— Yes, son?

— Why can't we go and live on the other side of the sea?

The father gave his son a stern look:

— Look at the sea, what do you see?

— Well,… I can see the horizon.

— And after it?

— Nothing.

— Exactly. There's nothing after the horizon. Is that where you want us to go?

His son did not say anything. The wind was blowing, and the seagulls cried as they flew over the sea.

— But daddy…, sometimes we see birds coming in from the horizon, don't we?

— They're able to fly above nothing, we're not.

The young boy did not look convinced. His father, irritated at his stubbornness (he felt he had seen more in his life), replied:

— Look at these waves, what do you see?

— They come and run aground in the sand.

— Exactly. In that case, in which direction are they moving?

— Towards the land.

— Why then do you want us to leave whereas the waves will keep on bringing us back towards land?

We can judge after seeing. But we can never be certain of seeing well or judging well.

| EPILOGUE |

Here is the sixty-ninth story. By way of conclusion, I wish to let you know how these short tales about compassion had an impact on my own life, and what prompted me to write them down and share them with you.

I am a doctor by profession. Herein lies the paradox of this book: my science-oriented training would naturally lead me to lean towards rationalism. The principles of compassion did not really fall under my way of life nor my medical training (at least not at the time I was undertaking my studies). However, in my medical work, I also come across patients with ailments related in part to mental issues.

I too, was once a victim of a heavily-laden lifestyle. At the beginning it had always been relatively easy for me to fall to sleep. Suddenly, one day, insomnia caught up with me.

It invaded my life and turned it upside down. This was the final breaking-point of my life after years of burdening myself with work and other worries.

It was at this point of my life when I encountered problems with falling asleep that I turned my attention to the subject of Compassion. I had tried many other methods with little success. I thus assumed a safety-release viewpoint as well as a patience and an acceptance mindset, whenever I could not get to sleep.

I have always been fascinated by the world of sleep and dreams. I have come across patients in my profession who have suffered for years due to lack of sleep; ever since I came to learn about the importance of nasal breathing for a good night's sleep.

In my opinion, sleep time is a very crucial moment in our lives, which unfortunately has been ignored in our modern societies. Most people have come to see it as a "waste of time". However, the effects and benefits of sleep have positive impacts on all aspects of our lives: health, vitality, mentality, memory, etc.

My research in this subject has led me to carry out studies on behaviors that encourage sleep. Little by little, I have tested, sorted, and selected the best "methods" for a peaceful, natural sleep. The most ideal is to associate reading positive stories with the principle of Compassion.

I recommend this to anyone looking for a peaceful night's sleep after a hectic and stressful day. These are all easy-to-read tales that require no effort and have no hidden meanings. The aim is to simply let each story to blend into your sleep and gradually develop your mind towards a more peaceful life.

Let them come to life in you. Fill your minds with positive stories that progressively create an impact in your lives.

Is it not said that the best advice comes in your sleep?

www.ingramcontent.com/pod-product-compliance
Ingram Content Group UK Ltd.
Pitfield, Milton Keynes, MK11 3LW, UK
UKHW021658190726
13853UKWH00001B/349